A Step-by-Step Guide to Conducting an Integrative Review

Coleen E. Toronto · Ruth Remington
Editors

A Step-by-Step Guide to Conducting an Integrative Review

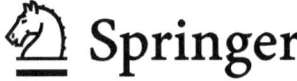 Springer

Editors
Coleen E. Toronto
School of Nursing
Curry College
Milton, MA
USA

Ruth Remington
Department of Nursing
Framingham State University
Framingham, MA
USA

ISBN 978-3-030-37503-4   ISBN 978-3-030-37504-1   (eBook)
https://doi.org/10.1007/978-3-030-37504-1

This Springer imprint is published by the registered company Springer Nature Switzerland AG
The registered company address is: Gewerbestrasse 11, 6330 Cham, Switzerland

Foreword

In nursing, we rely on integrative and other types of reviews for evidence to guide practice and reveal gaps in our knowledge that suggest further studies to be done. Reviews are critical to answer our questions about practice and how to care for patients. To make these important decisions, however, we need rigorous reviews that carefully and systematically search the literature, appraise studies, and synthesize findings. Without a strong methodology, the value of a review is questionable. Very few nurses and other health care providers are prepared to conduct an integrative review. Compounding this lack of preparation and understanding is the variety of terms used for reviews. There is no consistency in our definitions of the different types of reviews.

The focus of this book is on integrative reviews. These reviews are particularly valuable to nursing because they answer questions we have about practice, which guide the review, and involve a comprehensive search of the literature. In contrast to some types of reviews, in an integrative review, the quality of each of the studies is evaluated, and individual studies are then interpreted and synthesized into some meaningful conclusions to answer the questions and share new knowledge about the topic. This is what we need in nursing.

This is a must-read book for any nurse who is involved in evidence-based practice. It should be a required text for graduate students in nursing who need to develop skills in conducting integrative reviews as a basis for their scholarly projects and research. As prelicensure students learn about reviews, the book would be valuable for them too because it leads readers through each step of a review in a clear manner with examples. To move forward in nursing and health care, we need to understand how to conduct rigorous integrative reviews. This book explains the process, beginning with formulating questions to guide the review through the dissemination of the findings. There are no other books that focus on integrative reviews and provide the reader with a step-by-step process to use. This book by Drs. Toronto and Remington is a valuable resource for nurses, other health care providers, and nursing students at all levels.

Marilyn H. Oermann
Duke University School of Nursing
Durham, NC, USA

Preface

The integrative review is a frequent capstone project for graduate students and the basis for many doctoral projects. As educators, we have taught graduate students to conduct integrative reviews using book chapters and articles that covered integrative review methodology. These resources were limited and/or outdated and did not provide clear and practical advice on how to complete each step in the integrative review process. Due to this lack of resources, we would direct our students to look to the literature for published integrative reviews to help guide them when conducting their reviews; however, many reviews did not follow a consistent format and instead confused our students. These educational experiences were the impetus for our need to explore, in depth, the characteristics of published nurse-led reviews. We conducted a review to gain a better understanding of what a well-done review should look like and help us guide our students. Our review findings confirmed what we had been witnessing in the classroom with our students. There was much variation on how this type of review is conducted and published. Reviews often missed essential systematic steps to ensure rigor and decrease bias. An important implication from our published review was that there is a need for clear guidelines of what an integrative review is, and how it should be performed and reported. Research synthesis is difficult and time consuming. Because an integrative review is considered as actual research, it should be approached following established research methods involving well-defined steps. In this book, we provide the level of detail needed to systematically conduct an integrative review.

Milton, MA   Coleen E. Toronto
Framingham, MA   Ruth Remington

Contents

1 Overview of the Integrative Review 1
Coleen E. Toronto
  1.1 Introduction to Reviews 1
  1.2 Overview of Review Types.................................... 2
  1.3 Define Integrative Review Method............................ 4
  1.4 Barriers to Conducting an Integrative Review 5
  1.5 Systematic Approach 5
      1.5.1 Formulate Purpose and/or Review Question(s) 6
      1.5.2 Search and Select Literature Systematically.............. 6
      1.5.3 Quality Appraisal 7
      1.5.4 Analysis and Synthesis 7
      1.5.5 Discussion and Conclusion............................. 8
      1.5.6 Dissemination 8
  1.6 Conclusion 8
  References 8

2 Formulating Review Question 11
Karen Devereaux Melillo
  2.1 The Introduction Section of the IR............................ 12
  2.2 Defining Concepts and Variables 14
  2.3 Rationale for Conducting the Review.......................... 15
  2.4 Identify Purpose and/or Review Question(s) 16
  2.5 Formulate Inclusion and Exclusion Criteria.................... 17
  2.6 Identification of a Theoretical Framework 18
  2.7 Summary.. 19
  References 19

3 Searching Systematically and Comprehensively 21
Jane Lawless and Margaret J. Foster
  3.1 Librarian Support 22
  3.2 Search Organization and Reporting Strategies.................. 23
  3.3 Searching Considerations to Increase Rigor.................... 24
      3.3.1 Choosing Databases 24
      3.3.2 Terminology 25

       3.3.3   Nursing, Allied Health, and Medical Databases   25
       3.3.4   Interdisciplinary Databases   27
   3.4 Searching Systematically   27
       3.4.1   Natural and Controlled Language   28
       3.4.2   Combining Search Terms Using Boolean Logic   29
       3.4.3   Advanced Search Techniques   30
   3.5 Defining the Search Strategy   31
       3.5.1   Choosing Search Terms: Identifying Concepts   32
       3.5.2   Document the Search Process   33
       3.5.3   When Is the Database Search Process Complete?   34
   3.6 Screening for Study Selection   34
   3.7 Beyond Database Searching   36
       3.7.1   Gray Literature   37
       3.7.2   Conference Proceedings   37
       3.7.3   Dissertations/Theses   37
   3.8 Additional Methods of Searching   38
       3.8.1   Handsearching   38
       3.8.2   Citation/Related Article Searching   38
       3.8.3   Subject Experts   39
       3.8.4   Overall Gray Literature Resources   39
   3.9 Reporting the Search Strategy   39
       3.9.1   Managing the Collected Data   40
       3.9.2   Screening, Selecting, and Sorting   41
       3.9.3   Reporting Results of Screening and Selection   42
   3.10 Conclusion   42
   References   43

4 Quality Appraisal   45
   Ruth Remington
   4.1 Applying Inclusion Criteria   45
   4.2 Identifying Methodological Rigor   46
   4.3 Sources of Bias   46
   4.4 Validity   48
   4.5 Critical Appraisal Tools   48
       4.5.1   Design Specific Versus Generic   50
       4.5.2   Appraisal of Theoretical Literature   51
       4.5.3   Appraisal of Gray Literature   51
   4.6 Applicability of Results   52
       4.6.1   Reporting Guideline Versus Appraisal Tool   53
   4.7 Conclusion   53
   References   53

5 Analysis and Synthesis   57
   Patricia A. Dwyer
   5.1 Data Analysis and Synthesis   57

	5.2	Strategies for Data Analysis	58
		5.2.1 Creating a Data Matrix	58
		5.2.2 Data Analysis Methods	60
	5.3	Descriptive Results	68
	5.4	Synthesis	68
	References		69

6 Discussion and Conclusion 71
Coleen E. Toronto and Ruth Remington

	6.1	Writing the Discussion Section	72
		6.1.1 Audience	73
		6.1.2 Fundamental Structure	73
		6.1.3 Beginning the Discussion Section	73
	6.2	Interpretation of Findings	75
		6.2.1 Comparison to Background Literature	75
		6.2.2 Comparison to Theoretical Framework	76
		6.2.3 Comparison to Similar Research	77
		6.2.4 Unexpected Findings	77
	6.3	Implications	77
		6.3.1 Research	78
		6.3.2 Practice	78
		6.3.3 Education	79
		6.3.4 Policy	79
	6.4	Limitations	79
		6.4.1 Limitations of the Review	80
		6.4.2 Limitations of Literature Included in Reviews	80
	6.5	Conclusion	82
	6.6	Summary Points	82
	6.7	Conclusion	83
	References		83

7 Dissemination of the Integrative Review 85
Kristen A. Sethares

	7.1	The Integrative Review to Inform Practice, Program Planning, and Policy	85
	7.2	Writing Up the Integrative Review	86
		7.2.1 Manuscript Features	86
	7.3	Conference Presentation	91
		7.3.1 Submitting an Abstract	91
		7.3.2 Podium Presentation	91
		7.3.3 Poster Presentation	94
	7.4	Submitting the Integrative Review for Publication	96
		7.4.1 Selecting a Journal	96
		7.4.2 Preparing the Manuscript for Submission	100
		7.4.3 Manuscript Submission and Review	101

    7.5   New Approaches for Dissemination of Reviews 103
          7.5.1   News Media 103
          7.5.2   Social Media....................................... 104
    7.6   Future Needs to Update the Integrative Review................. 104
    References 105

Overview of the Integrative Review

1

Coleen E. Toronto

Contents

1.1	Introduction to Reviews.	1
1.2	Overview of Review Types.	2
1.3	Define Integrative Review Method.	4
1.4	Barriers to Conducting an Integrative Review.	5
1.5	Systematic Approach.	5
	1.5.1 Formulate Purpose and/or Review Question(s).	6
	1.5.2 Search and Select Literature Systematically.	6
	1.5.3 Quality Appraisal.	7
	1.5.4 Analysis and Synthesis.	7
	1.5.5 Discussion and Conclusion.	8
	1.5.6 Dissemination.	8
1.6	Conclusion.	8
References.		8

1.1 Introduction to Reviews

The purpose of a review is to summarize what is known about a topic and communicate the synthesis of literature to a targeted community. Before the advent of evidence-based practice, reviews were unsystematic, and there was no formal guidance on how to produce quality-synthesized evidence (Grant and Booth 2009). Conducting a review should parallel the steps a researcher undertakes when conducting a research study: formulation of a question(s) and collection and analysis of data (Polit and Beck 2018). In order for a review to be considered rigorous, a comprehensive method needs to be followed and reported.

C. E. Toronto (✉)
School of Nursing, Curry College, Milton, MA, USA
e-mail: ctoronto0712@curry.edu

© Springer Nature Switzerland AG 2020
C. E. Toronto, R. Remington (eds.), *A Step-by-Step Guide to Conducting an Integrative Review*, https://doi.org/10.1007/978-3-030-37504-1_1

This allows readers the ability to evaluate the reviewer's attempt to mitigate bias and, if desired, replicate the same review procedure and draw similar conclusions.

1.2   Overview of Review Types

With the expansion of evidence-based practice (EBP), the evolution of methods used in reviews has resulted in a wide spectrum of review types (Grant and Booth 2009; Whittemore et al. 2014). Due to the overlapping characteristics of the various review methods, confusion exists related to terminology and descriptions of each type (Aveyard and Bradbury-Jones 2019). The continuum for reviews begins with the most basic type, a narrative review, which summarizes selected literature on a topic and concludes with the most complex type; a systematic review of randomized control trials with meta-analysis, which collects; analyzes; appraises; and synthesizes randomized control studies to answer a single narrowly focused clinical question. To assist readers to understand the differences between the three most common types of reviews—narrative review, integrative review, and systematic review—descriptive summaries of each are presented in the following section and Table 1.1.

A *narrative review* does not follow a systematic method for locating and analyzing selected studies. It captures a "snapshot" of a clinical issue. Selected evidence found on a given topic often supports a reviewer's opinions or *a priori* assumptions of an issue (Conner 2014). Before systematic reviews emerged, this was how summarized evidence was presented (Coughlan and Cronin 2017).

The term *integrative review* is often used interchangeably with *systematic review*; however, there are distinct differences between them. The major differences are their purpose and scope, types of literature included, and time and resources needed to execute. An *integrative review* looks more broadly at a phenomenon of interest than a systematic review and allows for diverse research, which may contain theoretical and methodological literature to address the aim of the review. This approach supports a wide range of inquiry, such as defining concepts, reviewing theories, or analyzing methodological issues. Similar to the systematic review, it uses a systematic process to identify, analyze, appraise and synthesize all selected studies, but does not include statistical synthesis methods.

A *systematic review* has a single narrowly focused clinical question, usually formulated in a PICO (P = population, I = intervention, C = comparison, O = outcomes) format and may include meta-analysis. *Meta-analysis* is used to statistically synthesize data from several included studies to provide a single more precise estimate of the effectiveness of an intervention (Conner 2014). Both integrative and systematic reviews follow systematic steps, including asking a review question(s); identifying all potential electronic databases and sources to search; developing an explicit search strategy; screening titles, abstracts, and articles based on inclusion and exclusion criteria; and abstracting data from selected literature in a standardized format. Both use critical appraisal methods to assess the quality of each study, identify sources of bias, and synthesize data using transparent methods. These explicit

Table 1.1 Differences between the three common review types

	Narrative	Integrative	Systematic
Purpose	Provides an overview on a topic of inquiry for a research study, dissertation, or stand-alone review	Critical analysis of empirical, methodological, or theoretical literature, which draws attention to future research needs	Answers a single clinical question
Team member(s)	One or more reviewer	Two or more reviewers and librarian involvement recommended	Three or more reviewers includes librarian or information specialist and statistician if meta-analysis is performed.
A priori review protocol (plan)	No	No	Yes—protocol registration encouraged (PROSPERO, Cochrane Collaboration)
Review question	No	Broadly defined purpose and/or review question(s)	Single clinical question generally in the format of PICO P = population, I = intervention, C = comparison, O = outcomes
Established reporting guidelines	No	No	Yes (PRISMA reporting guidelines)
Timeline	2–6 months	6–12 months	12–24 months
Use of a systematic search methodology (allows for replication)	No	Yes	Yes
Sampling	Scholarly work on topic	Experimental/ nonexperimental research—may include theoretical and methodological literature	Experimental research
Eligibility (inclusion and exclusion)	No	Yes	Yes
Search flow diagram	No	Yes	Yes (PRISMA flow diagram)
Critical appraisal	No	Yes	Yes
Data extraction	No	Yes	Yes
Analysis and synthesis	Narrative analysis	Narrative and/or thematic analysis with descriptive and qualitative synthesis	Narrative analysis with descriptive and qualitative synthesis— may include quantitative synthesis (meta-analysis)
EBP Implications	No	Yes	Yes

methods reduce the chance for reviewers to only select literature that supports their own opinions or research hypotheses. Overall, systematic reviews take more time to complete and require more resources compared to narrative and integrative reviews. Before a reviewer selects a particular review method to follow to synthesize evidence, the breadth and depth of the review question(s) and scope of inquiry need to be considered (Gough et al. 2012).

Evidence-based care calls for the integration of best research evidence, clinical expertise, and values of the patient. The amount and complexity of evidence that healthcare professionals need to inform evidence-based practice (EBP) can be overwhelming. A rigorously conducted review can provide nurses and other healthcare disciplines a comprehensive update on a topic of interest or concern. A well-prepared review synthesizes many studies and can translate this evidence into practice sooner, less than the often cited 17 years (Morris et al. 2011).

Systematic reviews of randomized control trials (RCTs) using meta-analysis to determine the effectiveness of a healthcare intervention are considered the highest level of evidence in medicine and allows a clinician to make the best and most up-to-date healthcare decisions on interventions for treatment. There are many resources available for reviewers to use that provide guidance on how best to conduct and report a systematic review (Aromataris and Munn 2017; Higgins et al. 2019; Institute of Medicine 2011; Moher et al. 2009). The remainder of this chapter and book will focus on the less understood integrative review (IR) method; how is it defined, barriers in the use of this type of method, and the method's systematic process.

1.3   Define Integrative Review Method

An IR uses a broad approach and diverse sampling that include empirical or theoretical literature, or both (Cooper 1984). IRs provide synthesis on: (1) empirical research (review of quantitative and/or qualitative empirical studies on a particular topic), (2) methodological (review and analyses of designs and methodologies of different studies), and (3) theoretical (review of theories on a particular topic) (Whittemore et al. 2014; Soares et al. 2014).

An IR synthesizes research and draws conclusions from diverse sources on a topic. This enables the reviewer the ability to provide a more holistic understanding of a specific phenomenon. The IR method enables a reviewer to address: (1) the current state of evidence of a particular phenomenon, (2) the quality of the evidence, (3) gaps in the literature, and (4) identify the future steps for research and practice (Russell 2005). A well-prepared IR follows a systematic process and includes appraised and synthesized literature from diverse literatures to address phenomena relevant to a particular field of study (Soares et al. 2014; de Souza et al. 2010). Moreover, when appropriate, experts suggest using a theoretical framework to guide the IR process (Soares et al. 2014; Russell 2005; Denney and Tewksbury 2013; Torraco 2005). A broad conceptual definition of the IR has been provided, and attention to the differences between the IR method and other review methodologies is noted throughout this chapter and the remainder of the book.

1.4   Barriers to Conducting an Integrative Review

Methodological discourse of the IR method began to emerge in the 1980s in the fields of education, psychology, and nursing (Cooper 1982, 1984; Jackson 1980; Ganong 1987). Despite the high level of interest at that time, the evidence base for how best to conduct IRs remains limited, and no consistent set of acceptable standards or guidelines are available at this time for reviewers to consult. Slow development may be attributed to the need for combining diverse methodologies (experimental, nonexperimental research, and theoretical literature), which adds complexity for analysis, synthesis, and conclusion drawing (Whittemore and Knafl 2005).

The absence of formal guidelines for IRs had prompted several researchers in the field of nursing education to explore published IRs in order to gain a better understanding of how IRs are conducted. Researchers found the use of inconsistent review methods and lack of rigor in many reviews conducted by nurse reviewers (Hopia et al. 2016; Toronto et al. 2018).

While few articles address how to write an IR (Torraco 2005, 2016; Whittemore and Knafl 2005), the coverage in research textbooks on the process of conducting an IR is more limited and is often presented in a brief summary or chapter. In 1980, Jackson (1980) pointed out that the limited information on review methods found in textbooks presents an obstacle not only to novice student reviewers but also to experienced reviewers. Despite these barriers, IRs are frequently published internationally in high-impact nursing research journals supporting the utility of this type of review to inform evidence-based practice in nursing (Soares et al. 2014). A major reason for the popularity of the IR method in nursing is that it uses diverse data sources to investigate the complexity of nursing practice more broadly compared to a narrowly focused clinical question found in systematic reviews. Evidence produced from well-conducted IRs contributes to nursing knowledge by clarifying phenomena, which in turn informs nursing practice and clinical practice guidelines.

1.5   Systematic Approach

Both the systematic review and IR require a systematic approach that is transparent and rigorous. Cooper's widely used methodological approach for an IR has provided guidance for reviewers on how best to conduct an IR (Cooper 1982, 1984; Russell 2005; de Souza et al. 2010; Whittemore and Knafl 2005). This methodological approach consists of five stages to guide the design of an IR: (1) problem formulation stage, in which the broad purpose and review question(s) are clearly stated; (2) literature search stage, which uses a comprehensive and replicable search strategy to collect data; (3) data evaluation stage, in which the methodological quality and relevance of selected literature are appraised; (4) data analysis stage, which includes data abstraction, comparison, and synthesis; and (5) presentation stage, in which the interpretation of findings and implications for research; practice; and policy as well as the

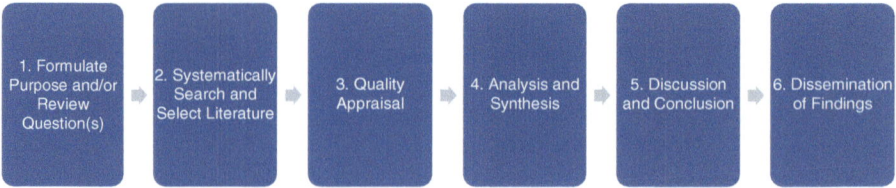

Fig. 1.1 The six steps of the integrative review process

limitations of the review are presented, and the importance of disseminating the findings is also addressed (Cooper 1984). Since its first debut, Cooper's five stages have been revisited, and variations have been proposed (de Souza et al. 2010; Whittemore and Knafl 2005). The IR process to be addressed in this book will follow Cooper's framework as a foundation when describing the key steps of the IR process. Figure 1.1 provides an example of the six steps of the IR process.

The following section will provide a summary of each step of the IR process: (1) formulation of a broad purpose and/or review question(s), (2) systematic search of the literature using predetermined criteria, (3) critical appraisal of selected research, (4) analysis and synthesis of literature, (5) discussion on new knowledge, and (6) dissemination plans of findings.

1.5.1 Formulate Purpose and/or Review Question(s)

The IR process begins with clearly identifying a problem from a gap in the literature.

The concepts of interest related to the research problem need to be clearly defined. The development of the background and significance for the research problem will provide justification for why the review is necessary or what is commonly referred to as the "so what" factor (relevance). Developing the purpose and/or review question(s) is an interactive and inductive process that takes place over time. It is critical that the review purpose and questions are broad and well defined as it informs the search criteria and data collection procedures used in the review (Whittemore and Knafl 2005; Oermann and Hays 2016).

1.5.2 Search and Select Literature Systematically

The literature search should be systematic in its approach and comprehensive using two or more methods, such as the use of multiple electronic databases and ancestry and hand search (the task of searching through peer-reviewed journals) methods. The purpose of comprehensive searches is to minimize biased conclusions in reviews (Whittemore 2007). A method used to improve the reporting of the search in an IR follows steps described in the Preferred Reporting Items for Systematic Reviews and Meta-Analyses (PRISMA) reporting guidelines (Moher et al. 2009).

It takes a significant amount of time to conduct an IR. To increase specificity and comprehensiveness of searches, a consultation with a librarian is advised. The librarian can assist with identifying effective search terms and how to save and manage searches utilizing a citation management system. Organization is critical to the success of conducting a search for a review. The purpose and/or review question(s) should be used as a guide when formulating inclusion and exclusion criteria to identify and manage selected articles. In addition to years of publications, study designs, and language of publications; limiters applied (i.e., peer reviewed), truncated terms and Boolean operators used, and date last search all require documentation. Reviewers should describe their search methods in such a way that it will allow another reviewer the ability to replicate or evaluate their search.

Effective inclusion and exclusion criteria will help to prevent a sample from becoming too wieldy or too small. An essential step in the study selection process is screening, which involves reviewing the citations resulting from a search and selecting those deemed relevant for full-text retrieval, and critical appraisal of the retrieved studies. All sampling decisions made need to be transparent and justified. A search flow diagram such as the PRISMA flow diagram assists with the reporting of the selection process of literature for the review sample (Moher et al. 2009). Initial screening entails screening titles and abstracts of potentially relevant literature using identified criteria. Then, the full text of the remaining literature is evaluated to determine the inclusion. The reviewer will next document this process and the reasons why an article was excluded in a search flow diagram.

1.5.3 Quality Appraisal

When conducting an IR, it is crucial to assess the quality or internal validity of the studies selected (Denney and Tewksbury 2013). The strength of a review's findings is reliant on the quality of studies included (Coughlan and Cronin 2017). A major difference from a narrative review is the assessment of quality in selected studies that occurs in an IR. The appraisal is one way a reviewer attempts to mitigate bias studies selected. There are many quality appraisal tools available to assist reviewers when assessing the methodological quality of a study.

1.5.4 Analysis and Synthesis

IRs require a narrative analysis and integration of a large amount of existing data to generate a new perspective on the topic of interest (Torraco 2016). It is a complex undertaking and requires transparent and credible methods (Whittemore 2007). Reviewers will need to extract data into matrices (tables) and analyze for similarities and differences (patterns) in relation to the stated review purpose or questions. These patterns are then synthesized. In this process, reviewers will need to move from mere facts related on a problem to a conceptual level of knowledge related to their inquiry.

1.5.5 Discussion and Conclusion

The discussion section of an IR is where reviewers write about what their review findings mean. Comparisons and contrasts are made of the findings of the review with background literature, and work of others. Recommendations and implications for research, practice, education, theory, and policy when applicable are made. Reviewers then comment on methodological limitations of their review. The conclusion will include a concise summary of their major findings and key contributions to the state of science.

1.5.6 Dissemination

Dissemination occurs when a reviewer communicates their synthesis of research to a targeted professional community. It has been proposed that IRs use the same format as primary research, which includes introduction, method, results, and discussion sections. The dissemination phase is the final step of the IR (Cooper 1984). The means for dissemination of the findings from an integrative literature review can occur via poster or podium presentations at professional conferences, peer-reviewed publication, news, and social media, and is essential to the development of a discipline's knowledge base.

1.6 Conclusion

Evidence-based practice requires synthesis of literature for nurses to keep up-to-date in practice. There are several common review methods used in healthcare, and it is important that nurses recognize the differences between each type. The IR is one method commonly published in nursing due to its broad focus and ability to address clinical issues in a holistic manner.

Presently, there are no consistent set of acceptable standards or guidelines available for how best to conduct IRs, which can impact the quality of review findings. Conducting rigorous IRs is necessary in order to produce strong evidence that informs nursing practice. The IR requires a systematic approach that is transparent and rigorous. The IR process covered in this book will include the following steps: (1) formulation of broad purpose and/or review question(s), (2) systematic search and selection of literature using predetermined criteria, (3) appraisal of quality of selected studies, (4) analysis and synthesis of literature, (5) discussion on new knowledge, and (6) dissemination of findings.

References

Aromataris E, Munn Z (eds) (2017) Joanna Briggs Institute reviewer's manual. The Joanna Briggs Institute. https://reviewersmanual.joannabriggs.org/

Aveyard H, Bradbury-Jones C (2019) An analysis of current practices in undertaking literature reviews in nursing: findings from a focused mapping review and synthesis. BMC Med Res Methodol 19:1. https://doi.org/10.1186/s12874-019-0751-7

Conner BT (2014) Demystifying literature reviews. Am Nurse Today 9(1):13–14

Cooper HM (1982) Scientific guidelines for conducting integrative research reviews. Rev Educ Res 52:291–302. https://doi.org/10.2307/1170314

Cooper HM (1984) The integrative research review: a systematic approach. SAGE Publications, Beverly Hills, CA, p 11

Coughlan M, Cronin P (2017) Doing a literature review in nursing, health and social care, 2nd edn. SAGE Publications, Thousand Oaks, CA, p 12

de Souza MT, da Silva MD, de Carvalho R (2010) Integrative review: what is it? How to do it? Einstein (São Paulo) 8(1):102–106. https://doi.org/10.1590/s1679-45082010rw1134

Denney AS, Tewksbury R (2013) How to write a literature review. J Crim Justice Educ 24(2):218–234. https://doi.org/10.1080/10511253.2012.730617

Ganong LH (1987) Integrative review of nursing research. Res Nurs Health 10(1):1–11

Gough D, Thomas J, Oliver S (2012) Clarifying differences between review designs and methods. Syst Rev 1:28. https://doi.org/10.1186/2046-4053-1-28

Grant MJ, Booth A (2009) A typology of reviews: an analysis of review types and associated methodologies. Health Inf Libr J 26:91–108. https://doi.org/10.1111/j.1471-1842.2009.00848.x

Higgins JPT, Thomas J, Chandler J, Cumpston M, Li T, Page MJ, Welch VA (eds) (2019) Cochrane handbook for systematic reviews of interventions version 6.0 (updated July 2019). Cochrane. www.training.cochrane.org/handbook

Hopia H, Latvala E, Liimatainen L (2016) Reviewing the methodology of an integrative review. Scand J Caring Sci 30:662–669. https://doi.org/10.1111/scs.12327

Institute of Medicine (2011) Finding what works in health care: standards for systematic reviews. The National Academies Press, Washington, DC. https://doi.org/10.17226/13059

Jackson GB (1980) Methods for integrative reviews. Rev Educ Res Rev 50:438–460. https://doi.org/10.2307/1170440

Moher D, Liberati A, Tetzlaff J, Altman DG (2009) Preferred reporting items for systematic reviews and meta-analyses: the PRISMA statement. J Clin Epidemiol 62(10):1006–1012. https://doi.org/10.1016/j.jclinepi.2009.06.005

Morris ZS, Wooding S, Grant J (2011) The answer is 17 years, what is the question: understanding time lags in translational research. J R Soc Med 104(12):510–520. https://doi.org/10.1258/jrsm.2011.110180

Oermann MH, Hays JC (2016) Writing for publication in nursing, 3rd edn. Springer, New York, NY, p 136

Polit DF, Beck CT (2018) Essentials of nursing research: appraising evidence for nursing practice, 9th edn. Wolters Kluwer, Philadelphia, p 96

Russell CL (2005) An overview of the integrative research review. Prog Transplant 15(1):8–13. https://doi.org/10.7182/prtr.15.1.0n13660r26g725kj

Soares CB, Hoga LAK, Peduzzi M, Sangaleti C, Yonekura T, Silva D (2014) Integrative review: concepts and methods used in nursing. Rev Esc Enferm USP 48(2):329–339. https://doi.org/10.1590/s0080-623420140000200020

Toronto CE, Quinn B, Remington R (2018) Characteristics of reviews published in nursing literature: a methodological review. ANS Adv Nurs Sci 41(1):30–40. https://doi.org/10.1097/ANS.0000000000000180

Torraco RJ (2005) Writing integrative literature reviews: guidelines and examples. Hum Resour Dev Rev. SAGE Publications 4(3):356–367. https://doi.org/10.1177/1534484305278283

Torraco RJ (2016) Writing integrative literature reviews: using the past and present to explore the future. Hum Resour Dev Rev 15(4):404–428. https://doi.org/10.1177/1534484316671606

Whittemore R (2007) Rigour in integrative reviews. In: Webb C, Roe B (eds) Reviewing research evidence for nursing practice: in systematic reviews. Blackwell Publishing, Malden, MA, p 151

Whittemore R, Chao A, Jang M, Minges KE, Park C (2014) Methods for research synthesis: an overview. Heart Lung 43(5):453–461. https://doi.org/10.1016/j.hrtlng.2014.05.014

Whittemore R, Knafl K (2005) The integrative review: updated methodology. J Adv Nurs 52(5):546–553. https://doi.org/10.1111/j.1365-2648.2005.03621.x

Formulating Review Question

2

Karen Devereaux Melillo

Contents

2.1	The Introduction Section of the IR...	12
2.2	Defining Concepts and Variables..	14
2.3	Rationale for Conducting the Review..	15
2.4	Identify Purpose and/or Review Question(s)...	16
2.5	Formulate Inclusion and Exclusion Criteria...	17
2.6	Identification of a Theoretical Framework..	18
2.7	Summary...	19
References...		19

Previously, the reader was introduced to what distinguishes the integrative review (IR) from narrative and systematic reviews. In this chapter, the focus is on a clear identification of the gaps in knowledge as it pertains to the phenomenon of interest that will be addressed in the integrative review. This is accomplished by the development of key concepts and identification of the target population, which leads to the formulation of inclusion and exclusion criteria, which guide the literature search for the review.

One of the distinguishing aspects of the integrative review is that the sampling for an IR may include experimental and nonexperimental (empirical) and theoretical literature, for inclusion in integrative reviews. The *Publication Manual of the American Psychological Association* (2010) defines empirical literature as "reports of original research"; theoretical literature as that which "draws on existing research

K. D. Melillo (✉)
University of Massachusetts Lowell, Solomont School of Nursing, Lowell, MA, USA
e-mail: Karen_Melillo@uml.edu

© Springer Nature Switzerland AG 2020   11
C. E. Toronto, R. Remington (eds.), *A Step-by-Step Guide to Conducting an Integrative Review*, https://doi.org/10.1007/978-3-030-37504-1_2

literature to advance theory" (American Psychological Association 2010, p. 10). The findings from this preliminary background literature review could then support proceeding with the development of a review purpose or review questions to address the phenomenon of interest.

2.1   The Introduction Section of the IR

The introduction of the IR provides the background and rationale for conducting the review. The introduction and background direct the reader from the very broad general topic to the IR's specific approach to the issue being reviewed and ultimately synthesized (Denney and Tewksbury 2013). The introduction will usually start with a brief summary of existing knowledge and previous research on the topic under consideration. In addition to research, theoretical literature may help to define concepts. Previous reviews may further the development of the topic and justify the need for proceeding with a new review, while at the same time helping to identify a gap in current knowledge. Moreover, gray literature (unpublished technical or research reports), which may or may not be peer reviewed, can be used to support the development of the topic of inquiry in the introduction. The introduction might also include information from national organizations, professional associations, or government agencies where position papers and statistical data on prevalence, incidence, and current evidence-based practice guidelines may be referenced.

A scientific paper typically has four parts, the introduction, methods, results, and discussion, also known as the IMRaD structure. The introduction starts with a review of the phenomenon of interest in the broadest context to provide the reader with a background to the topic. Once the conceptual overview is complete, the introduction moves into the more specific description of how the phenomenon is to be addressed in the review, the setting or context, and the population being studied. Any gap in the literature is then presented and should be explicitly described. The purpose and/or review question(s) follows at the end of the introduction (Suramanyam 2013). The purpose describes the goal of the review, or why the review is being conducted. The review question(s) succinctly identifies what the review proposes to answer and suggests how it might contribute to a better understanding of the phenomenon of interest (Aveyard 2014).

A model known as the hourglass model (Jirge 2017; Schulte 2003) is an approach to writing scientific papers. It has been suggested as being helpful in conceptualizing the integrative review process as well. Visually, the top of the hourglass is quite broad. For the IR, this is where the introduction identifies a broad problem area, related concepts, and the research history and states the importance of the topic in general. As the top of the hourglass narrows, so does the focus of the introduction to the specific purpose statement and/or review questions. The method proposed to answer the review question(s) is the most specific part of the introduction represented by the narrowest part of the top half of the hourglass (Fig. 2.1).

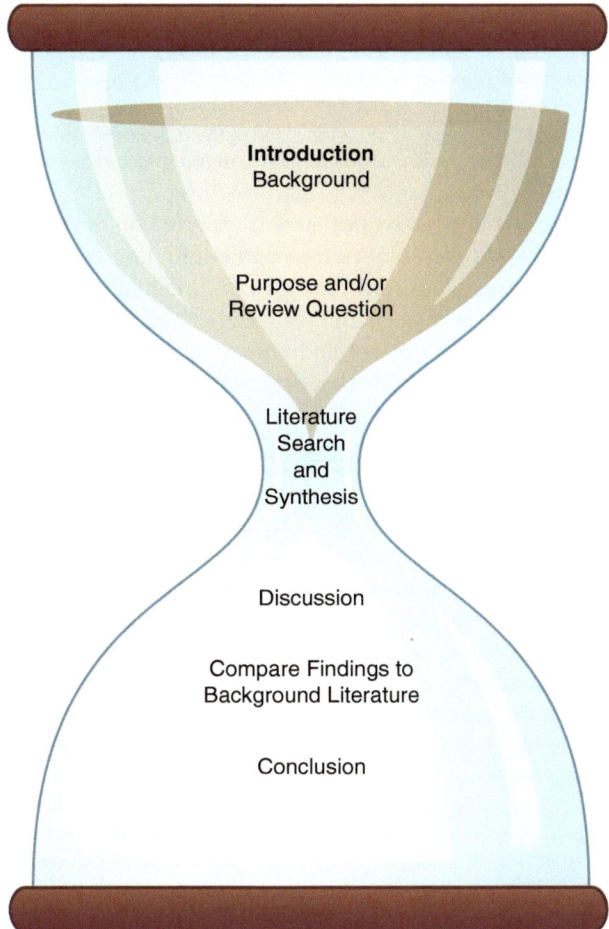

Fig. 2.1 Hourglass model

The introduction identifies and describes the phenomenon to be investigated; operationalizes the phenomenon, population, and context; and summarizes relevant research to present the gap in the literature that the review is to fill (Hudson-Barr 2004). In an IR exploring self-efficacy for management of symptoms and symptom distress, White and colleagues (White et al. 2019) identify the phenomenon to be investigated as follows:

> Self-management of symptoms affects the cost of health care through treatment-related services, hospitalizations, and use of the healthcare system, and it can reduce symptom distress and increase QOL. Self-efficacy for symptom management is a predictor of outcomes for populations with chronic diseases and is important for managing the complex challenges of cancer treatment. (p. 113)

They then operationalized the phenomenon, population, and setting for the review by specifying how the concept of self-efficacy is to be used in the review, what the population of interest is, and the context for the review.

> …self-efficacy for management of symptoms and symptom distress in adults with cancer, particularly those undergoing hematopoietic stem cell transplantation. (p. 113)

The importance of previous work that was reported on the topic area should be discussed, and any unanswered questions and conflicting or challenging findings should be described (Hudson-Barr 2004). In an integrative review of the experiences of internationally educated nurses (IEN) and their transition to practice (TTP) in the United States, Ghazel and colleagues (2019) highlighted an unanswered question regarding the transition experiences of IENs working in the United States.

> It remains unclear whether the transition experiences of IENs are similar among different source countries and receiving countries, and it has yet to be summarized what TTP experiences exist for IENs working solely in the United States. (p. 5)

The IR introduction section concludes with the purpose and/or review question(s) that the IR will address (Patriotta 2017). The review question(s) guides the literature search and data collection. An IR on the barriers that nurses face in providing evidence-based practice (EBP), Middlebrooks and colleagues (2016) posed a question to guide further exploration of the topic. The question identified the phenomenon of interest (barriers to EBP), the population (clinically based nurses), and the context (2004–2015).

> The question guiding this integrative review was: What strategies have been implemented to reduce individual barriers to EBP of clinically based nurses, as reported in the literature reviewed from 2004 to 2015? (p. 399)

2.2   Defining Concepts and Variables

Conducting an integrative review begins with the identification of a topic or concept of interest (Beyea and Nicoll 1998; Broome 2000). Because the reviewer will be spending considerable time developing the integrative review, the topic should be one that stimulates curiosity and is meaningful to the reviewer and the profession.

It is important to minimize any ambiguity in the IR by clearly describing what is meant by the variables and how they will be used in the review. The conceptual and operational definitions of variables to be examined need to be developed. The conceptual definition describes what the concept means, whereas the operational definition describes the concept in observable and measurable terms as used in the review. For example, a reviewer is interested in studying the concept of stress among college students. The conceptual definition of stress could be "a particular relationship between the person and the environment that is appraised by the person as taxing or exceeding his or her resources and endangering his or her well-being" (Lazarus and Folkman 1984, p. 19). This could be operationalized for the review as the level of the stress hormone cortisol or a score on the Daily Hassles and Uplifts Scale. Similarly, the concept of illness may be interpreted as sickness, or complaint, or ailment or disorder, all similar instances of illness, but if the review is to deal with heart failure, illness should be operationalized as "heart failure." The definition of the concept should be made explicit because it will influence what literature is retrieved for analysis and what information is extracted from the identified sample (Broome), and ultimately delineate the scope of the review.

An example of a conceptual definition and an operational definition of coping can be found in the IR conducted by Ruckholdt and colleagues (2019). In the IR on coping by family members of critically ill hospitalized patients, coping was conceptually defined using the definition of Lazarus and Folkman as "a person's cognitive and behavioural efforts in response to stressors that determine how those stressors will affect physical and emotional well-being" (p. 41). Coping was operationally defined for the review as the coping strategies that adults identified after the admission of their family member to the ICU, as identified in the literature.

Before undertaking the IR, the reviewer may choose to reach out to notable scholars of prior reviews or authors of primary research related to the phenomenon of interest. Contact names and emails of corresponding authors are often provided in peer-reviewed journal articles. With a clear purpose in mind and having conducted the preliminary review, the reviewer can introduce themselves and indicate why they are reaching out. Specifically, the novice reviewer may be unaware of current in press journal articles, position papers in preparation, or additional reviews/research that would provide important background for conducting, or choosing to conduct, the IR. Nurse scholars and authors are most amenable to offering input and suggestions, provided the details of the request are succinct.

2.3 Rationale for Conducting the Review

Before the IR takes place, a preliminary review of the literature is conducted to support the need for the review. This will often take the form of an exploration that examines, or asks, "what is out there?" regarding a phenomenon of interest. But how does one determine whether an integrative review is the best method to address the knowledge gap, versus conducting another type of review? If the purpose or review question is broadly focused, versus narrowly defined, this supports that an IR is the way to proceed. An example of a broad focus in a review question in an integrative review is "What are the TTP (transition to practice) experiences of IENs (internationally educated nurses) working in the United States from 2000 to 2018?" (Ghazal et al. 2019, p. 399). Whereas a focus, not appropriate for an IR, would be a narrowly defined intervention. A PICO (Population, Intervention, Comparison, Outcome) question would be an example of a question that would be more appropriate for a systematic review. In the following example, in obese adults (P), does weight loss (I) compared with a proton pump inhibitor (C) better reduce symptoms of gastroesophageal reflux (O)? The focus is narrow, dealing with a particular intervention, and quantitative research is likely the only literature that would address the effect of this intervention.

Because the purposes of reviews may differ, it is important that the authors identify the purpose of their review early on, soon after the gap in the literature is identified (Torraco 2016). There are a number of purposes to conduct an integrative review, including to review, critique, and update what is known or unknown about the phenomenon of interest, to identify gaps in the literature about the phenomenon, to reconceptualize the phenomenon, and to critique and synthesize literature to determine the state of the science related to the phenomenon of interest (Torraco 2016; Krainovich-Miller 2017).

2.4 Identify Purpose and/or Review Question(s)

The IR review question(s) allows one to explore issues relevant to nursing (Russell 2005). Choosing the topic for the IR is the first step. Being clear to have this be a relevant, well-defined, and broadly focused topic is vital. Completing an IR can take 6 or more months. It is important that the IR is feasible within the time line available, particularly if this is a student assignment within an academic course, where time frame and resources may be limited.

To develop a clear, focused, and relevant review question(s), the reviewer should consider the "who, what, where, when, why, and how" questions related to the topic. These questions will also provide the details necessary for identifying inclusion and exclusion criteria and for the subsequent review of the literature. Keep in mind the purpose of the review (why the review is being undertaken) and the problem formulation/rationale for conducting the review (what the review is about) in developing the review question(s).

Review questions are directly linked to the problem formulation—that area of concern where there is a gap in knowledge (Fisch and Block 2018). Within each review question, variables or concepts of interest are identified. Doing so will provide the basis for the specified inclusion and exclusion criteria for the study sample.

In posing a review question, avoid questions that can be answered by "yes" or "no." For example, the question guiding the review was "do nursing students experience stress?" would probably be answered with a "yes" by many people and does not leave much room for synthesis or analysis, so there is no need to read the whole review. However, if the question was "what strategies do nursing students employ to cope with stress?," there are many possible explanations that the review could provide.

Having clearly stated review question(s), based on a carefully developed introduction and background, then sets the stage for the undertaking of the IR. Thus, the review question(s) becomes a critical component of the introduction section (Evans 2007).

2.5 Formulate Inclusion and Exclusion Criteria

By crafting clear review question(s), the reviewer(s) is able to identify inclusion and exclusion criteria to refine the sample of literature. Stated simply, inclusion criteria are characteristics that literature must have in order to be included. Exclusion criteria are the characteristics that would make a study ineligible to be included in the review. Because integrative reviews address broad questions, it is likely that a search will retrieve a large volume of literature. Application of inclusion and exclusion criteria can make the amount of literature that needs to be screened more manageable and help to identify relevant papers for the review. Explicit criteria can help to minimize the risk of bias and allow the reader to make a judgment about the validity of the review (Evans 2007). In an IR about pediatric pain management in the emergency department, Williams and colleagues (2019) provided an example of explicit criteria for the selection of literature to include in the review:

> Studies were considered if the population was deemed to be paediatric; a strict age range was not applied. In the spirit of an integrative review, this enabled inclusion of several significant studies which may have otherwise been excluded. Interventions of interest were those that aimed to improve emergency department paediatric pain management at a systems or organisational level… Outcomes of interest specifically related to pain management including: time to analgesia, provision of analgesia, reassessment of pain, repeat analgesia, reduction in pain score, child/parent satisfaction, parental knowledge and clinician knowledge. There were no date limitations specified. Studies were excluded if they related to a strictly adult population, compared or measured effectiveness of specific medications, focused on a specific chronic illness (e.g., sickle cell disease), or investigated procedure-related pain. There was no restriction on study design. (p. 11)

Explicit inclusion criteria also help to prevent the influence of confounding variables. All decisions about literature to include or exclude should be justified and documented in the methods to demonstrate that an unbiased process was followed. Examples of components of the inclusion criteria to refine the search may include the following:

- Types of studies or literature.
- The phenomenon under investigation.
- The characteristics of the population being studied.
- Publication language.
- Time period covered by the review and its justification.
- Setting (Garrard 2014; Stern et al. 2014).

A common error regarding inclusion and exclusion criteria is using the same variable to define both the inclusion and exclusion criteria. For example, if an inclusion criterion is that the subjects are 65 or more years of age, it is not necessary to state an exclusion criterion of less than 65 years of age. If the studies are to be excluded for methodological quality, this should be stated with a clear description of the measures used to determine acceptable methodological quality. The reviewer should make sure that the inclusion and exclusion criteria are aligned with the review purpose and/or question(s).

2.6   Identification of a Theoretical Framework

Several authors have advocated that a theoretical framework or conceptual model guides and organizes integrative reviews (Denney and Tewksbury 2013; Torraco 2016; Fisch and Block 2018; Soares et al. 2014). If a theoretical framework is used to guide the review, an explanation of how this framework will be organizing the integrative review should be included. There needs to be a clear connection between the theory and its concepts to the review purpose, design, methods, and presentation of the results. All aspects of the review should connect to the theoretical framework thereby serving as a structure or framework for the review.

Not all IRs are conducted within the context of an established theoretical framework. In many IRs, a theoretical framework or conceptual model is not specified. However, in some IRs, the theory itself could serve as the basis for the review. For example, the theory of unpleasant symptoms (TOUS) (Blakeman 2019) guided the conduct of an IR, which explored how other researchers used it in the methodological design and analysis of symptom research, and to identify implications for further development of the theory. The review was structured around the three major concepts, the symptom, factors influencing the symptom, and performance outcomes. The conclusion was that the TOUS is helpful in understanding the multidimensional nature of many symptoms and can serve as a model for development of interventions. The authors recommended the need to further explore the symptom experience.

Another example of the use of a theoretical framework to structure an IR is Watson's Theory of Human Caring Science in an IR that explored the phenomenon of caring in the nurse–patient relationship through the caritas lens. The theory was integrated throughout the review, and the results were displayed within the 10 Caritas Processes (Settecase-Wu 2018).

Gough, Thomas, and Oliver (2012) point out that theoretical assumptions will underlie the choices made in operationalizing the review question. An example of how theoretical assumptions operationalize the review question (and subsequent choice of inclusion and exclusion criteria) is a review conducted by Cicero and colleagues (2019). In response to a call from the National Academy of Medicine for more research addressing the disparities that transgender adults experience in healthcare, these authors conducted an IR guided by the gender affirmation framework. The framework is composed of four constructs: social gender affirmation, medical gender affirmation, psychological gender affirmation, and legal gender affirmation among transgender adults. These constructs were previously demonstrated to influence healthcare utilization among this group of individuals. The framework guided the selection of the search terms used to identify the sample of studies evaluated in the review, as well as the identification of the inclusion and exclusion criteria. Results of the review were organized according to the four constructs.

2.7 Summary

This chapter focused on the development of an introduction section of an IR. It began with the general topic background and identification of what is known and what gaps in knowledge may exist. A rationale for conducting the review will be articulated based on a preliminary review of what is known and not known. Additionally, if a theoretical framework has been introduced, the explanation of how this framework will guide the integrative review should be included. The concepts and variables are then defined. In the process of defining the concepts and variables, inclusion and exclusion criteria are then delineated. After the purpose and/or review question(s) is clearly articulated, the reviewer will then determine whether an integrative review is the method of choice.

References

American Psychological Association (2010) The publication manual of the American Psychological Association, 6th edn. Author, Washington, DC. 272 p

Aveyard H (2014) Doing a literature review in health and social care: a practical guide, 3rd edn. McGraw-Hill, Maidenhead

Beyea SC, Nicoll LH (1998) Writing an integrative review. AORN J 67(4):877–880

Blakeman JR (2019) An integrative review of the theory of unpleasant symptoms. J Adv Nurs: 946–961. https://doi.org/10.1111/jan.13906

Broome ME (2000) Integrative literature reviews for the development of concepts. In: Rodgers BL, Knafl KA (eds) Concept development in nursing: foundations, techniques and applications, 2nd edn. WB Saunders, Philadelphia, pp 231–250

Cicero EC, Reisner SL, Silva SG, Merwin EI, Humphreys JC (2019) Health care experiences of transgender adults: an integrated mixed research literature review. Adv Nurs Sci 42(2): 123–138. https://doi.org/10.1097/ANS.0000000000000256

Denney AS, Tewksbury R (2013) How to write a literature review. J Crim Justice Educ 24(2): 102–106. https://doi.org/10.1080/10511253.2012.730617

Evans D (2007) Overview of methods. In: Webb C, Roe B (eds) Reviewing research evidence for nursing practice: in systematic reviews. Blackwell Publishing, Malden, MA, pp 137–148

Fisch C, Block J (2018) Six tips for your (systematic) literature review in business and management research. Manag Rev Q 68:103–106. https://doi.org/10.1007/s11302-018-0142.x

Garrard J (2014) Health sciences literature review made easy: the matrix method, 4th edn. Jones & Bartlett Learning, Burlington, MA

Ghazal LV, Ma C, Squires A (2019) Transition-to-US practice experiences of internationally educated nurses: an integrative review. West J Nurs Res. https://doi.org/10.1177/0193945919860855

Gough D, Thomas J, Oliver S (2012) Clarifying differences between research reviews and methodologies. Syst Rev 1:28–38. https://doi.org/10.1186/s13643-019-1089-2

Hudson-Barr D (2004) How to read a research article. J Spec Pediatr Nurs 9(2):70–72. https://doi.org/10.1111/j.1088-145X.2004.00070.x

Jirge PR (2017) Preparing and publishing a scientific manuscript. J Hum Reprod Sci 10(1):3–9. https://doi.org/10.4103/jhrs.JHRS_36_17

Krainovich-Miller B (2017) Gathering and appraising the literature. In: Wood LB, Haber J (eds) Nursing research: methods and critical appraisal for evidence-based practice, 9th edn. Elsevier, Mosby, St. Louis, MO, pp 45–65

Lazarus RS, Folkman S (1984) Stress appraisal and coping. Springer, New York

Middlebrooks R, Carter-Templeton H, Mund AR (2016) Effect of evidence-based practice programs on individual barriers of workforce nurses: an integrative review. J Contin Educ Nurs 47(9):398–406. https://doi.org/10.3928/00220124-20160817-06

Patriotta G (2017) Crafting papers for publication: novelty and convention in academic writing [Editorial]. J Manag Stud 54(5):747–759. https://doi.org/10.1111/joms.12280

Ruckholdt M, Tofler GH, Randall S, Buckley T (2019) Coping by family members of critically ill hospitalized patients: an integrative review. Int J Nurs Stud 97:40–54. https://doi.org/10.1016/j.ijnurstu.2019.04.016

Russell CL (2005) An overview of the integrative research review. Prog Transplant 15:8–13. https://doi.org/10.1177/152692480501500102

Schulte B (2003) Scientific writing and the scientific methodology: parallel hourglass structure in form and content. Am Biol Teach 65(8):591–594

Settecase-Wu C (2018) Caring in the nurse-patient relationship through the caritas lens an integrative review. Revista Cultura del Cuidado 15(2):34–66. https://doi.org/10.18041/1794-5232/cultrua.2018v15n2.5111

Soares CB, Hoga LA, Peduzzi M, Sangaleti C, Yonekura T, Silva DR (2014) Integrative review: concepts and methods used in nursing. Rev Esc Enferm USP 48(2):329–339. https://doi.org/10.1590/S0080-623420140000200020

Stern C, Jordan Z, McArthur A (2014) Developing the review question and inclusion criteria. Am J Nurs 114(4):53–56. https://doi.org/10.1097/01.NAJ.0000445689.67800.86

Suramanyam RV (2013) Art of reading a journal article: methodically and effectively. J Oral Maxillofac Pathol 17(1):65–70. https://doi.org/10.4103/0973-029X.110733

Torraco J (2016) Writing integrative literature reviews: using the past and present to explore the future. Hum Resour Dev Rev 15(4):404–428. https://doi.org/10.1177/1534484316671606

White LL, Cohen MZ, Berger AM, Kupzyk AZ, Bierman PJ (2019) Self-Efficacy for management of symptoms and symptom distress in adults with cancer: an integrative review. Oncol Nurs Forum 46:113–128

Williams S, Keogh S, Douglas C. (2019) Improving paediatric pain management in the emergency department: an integrative literature review. Int J Nurs Stud 94:9–20. https://doi.org/10.1016/j.ijnurstu2019.02.017

Searching Systematically and Comprehensively

Jane Lawless and Margaret J. Foster

Contents

3.1   Librarian Support... 22
3.2   Search Organization and Reporting Strategies............................. 23
3.3   Searching Considerations to Increase Rigor................................ 24
     3.3.1   Choosing Databases.. 24
     3.3.2   Terminology.. 25
     3.3.3   Nursing, Allied Health, and Medical Databases................. 25
     3.3.4   Interdisciplinary Databases..................................... 27
3.4   Searching Systematically... 27
     3.4.1   Natural and Controlled Language............................... 28
     3.4.2   Combining Search Terms Using Boolean Logic................. 29
     3.4.3   Advanced Search Techniques.................................... 30
3.5   Defining the Search Strategy.. 31
     3.5.1   Choosing Search Terms: Identifying Concepts.................. 32
     3.5.2   Document the Search Process.................................... 33
     3.5.3   When Is the Database Search Process Complete?................ 34
3.6   Screening for Study Selection.. 34
3.7   Beyond Database Searching.. 36
     3.7.1   Gray Literature... 37
     3.7.2   Conference Proceedings.. 37
     3.7.3   Dissertations/Theses... 37
3.8   Additional Methods of Searching... 38
     3.8.1   Handsearching... 38
     3.8.2   Citation/Related Article Searching.............................. 38
     3.8.3   Subject Experts.. 39
     3.8.4   Overall Gray Literature Resources.............................. 39
3.9   Reporting the Search Strategy.. 39

J. Lawless (✉)
Curry College, Milton, MA, USA
e-mail: jlawless@curry.edu

M. J. Foster
Texas A&M University, College Station, TX, USA
e-mail: margaretfoster@tamu.edu

© Springer Nature Switzerland AG 2020
C. E. Toronto, R. Remington (eds.), *A Step-by-Step Guide to Conducting an Integrative Review*, https://doi.org/10.1007/978-3-030-37504-1_3

    3.9.1   Managing the Collected Data... 40
    3.9.2   Screening, Selecting, and Sorting... 41
    3.9.3   Reporting Results of Screening and Selection.................................... 42
3.10 Conclusion... 42
References.. 43

Information is gathered at different stages of the integrative review (IR) process, including background information for formulating the question, and to support analysis and discussion. This chapter will focus on searching for, and identifying experimental; nonexperimental; and theoretical literature, which will be screened for inclusion or exclusion in the IR sample.

The IR process should include a clearly documented and comprehensive literature search, defining in detail all databases, search terms, limiters, eligibility (inclusion/exclusion), and criteria used, and describing any additional search methods (Cooper 1982; Whittemore and Knafl 2005). The search process for the systematic review has formal search guidelines and standards, which are clearly articulated; reviewed; and evaluated. However, the IR search process has been inconsistently described through articles and book chapters (Torraco 2005, 2016; Russell 2005; Soares et al. 2014; Hopia et al. 2016). The IR search process reflects the nature of the purpose and/or review questions addressed, which tends to be broader than the systematic review question, and draws its strategies from writings on knowledge synthesis and literature review, including systematic review.

3.1 Librarian Support

Reviewing published IRs reveals how librarians can support the search process (Coyne et al. 2018; Harstäde et al. 2018; Tobiano et al. 2015), and how librarians can play a valuable role (Middlebrooks et al. 2016). Librarians have experience building searches, identifying documentation tools, and organizing results. Working with a librarian helps to decrease the risk of bias by supporting a thorough and comprehensive search process (Evans 2007; Cooper et al. 2018). Bias is defined as any tendency that prevents unprejudiced consideration of a question (Pannucci and Wilkins 2010). There are different types of bias that can occur at different stages of the review process, which will be discussed in later sections of the book.

Many steps in the search process may be familiar to students and reviewers, but because the IR process requires documentation of each step, several steps benefit from more than one perspective. Working with a librarian can support rigor in a review, especially for a reviewer who is conducting the review alone. Although the process for developing the IR review question was addressed earlier, it should be remembered that preliminary searching may suggest revisions in the review question(s), and in that sense, the relationship between the review question(s) and the search strategy is a dynamic one. It is not unusual for sample searches to further define the question(s) and the eligibility (inclusion/exclusion) criteria. Engagement with search results may impact how the question(s) is finally articulated.

3.2   Search Organization and Reporting Strategies

A librarian can be helpful with recommending tools for literature organization. The reviewer is advised to consider how to document information described below *before* beginning the search process. Many of these topics will be discussed in more depth later in the chapter.

- Database selection benefits from discussion with a librarian. Depending on the nature of the IR review question, there may be relevant databases outside the normal scope of the reviewer's experience that should be considered (more information is found in Sect. 3.3.1). The names of selected databases, and the reasons why they were selected, can be saved in an Excel spreadsheet, a Word document, or other software application.
- Database searches should be saved, so search methods can be thoroughly described in the review, and potentially replicated. Searches can be saved in EBSCO, Ovid, PubMed, and many other databases, and while processes may be similar, they also may vary considerably. Tutorials (usually in video, PDF, or PowerPoint format) are helpful, and can be found through a Google search, such as "saving searches in CINAHL."
- Search results should be saved in an organized manner, so they can be screened for inclusion in the final review. For this purpose, citation management software (sometimes called bibliographic software applications) is helpful. Some require either an individual or institutional subscription; others are available at no cost.
- Search methods and results for gray literature (i.e., literature not controlled by commercial publishers, such as conference proceedings, clinical trials, dissertations/theses) can also be saved in citation management software. Although databases can automatically export to citation management software, many "gray" resources can be entered manually. Gray literature search methods will be discussed in more detail later in this chapter.
- Screening literature requires documentation that can be accomplished using citation management software, review software, or an Excel spreadsheet matrix.
- The IR search process will be reported in detail. This is done using the following:
  - A narrative description of all information sources, including databases, that were used; limiters used to narrow search results, such as year of publication, language, and publication status; and search terms used.
  - A search diagram format that depicts the flow of information through different phases of the review. PRISMA (Preferred Reporting Items for Systematic Reviews and Meta-Analyses) is an example of a reporting model that provides both a checklist and a search flow diagram that can be adapted for IR use (Moher et al. 2009). The PRISMA Flow Diagram (2015) will be discussed in later sections of this chapter.

3.3   Searching Considerations to Increase Rigor

Although recognized guidelines exist for conducting and reporting (PRISMA Flow Diagram 2015) systematic reviews and scoping reviews, IR searching guidelines have not been similarly formalized. Researchers who have studied IR methodology recommend that an IR includes a comprehensive search, one that captures as much literature pertaining to the topic as possible (Evans 2007; Whittemore 2007) and includes multiple strategies (Whittemore and Knafl 2005), such as searching more than one electronic databases to find peer-reviewed articles; searching the gray literature to find unpublished research and theoretical literature, which may not be included in electronic databases; and handsearching relevant journals and reference lists. Such a broad-based approach will help the reviewer to minimize bias and retrieve as much relevant literature as possible.

Because no single database indexes all relevant literature, searching only one database would result in the inclusion of a limited representation of studies/results. In other words, an IR search should go beyond CINAHL, and should utilize more than one or two search terms or phrases. Searching multiple databases contributes to a more comprehensive and rigorous review (Whittemore 2007; Higgins et al. 2019; Ganong 1987; Cooper 1998). Working with a librarian to select databases helps to identify useful sources that may be unfamiliar to the reviewer, another method to make the review more comprehensive and avoid bias.

3.3.1   Choosing Databases

Selecting databases for an IR can be a daunting task. The reviewer should be willing to move beyond familiar databases and consider new ones, documenting which databases were chosen and why. Fowler identified questions the reviewer should consider (Fowler 2017) when selecting databases for their review:

- Are the topics in the research (review) question covered in the database? CINAHL includes nursing and allied health publications; however, databases that include literature of other disciplines are suggested.
- What types of sources are indexed? IR can include research (experimental or nonexperimental) and theoretical literature. Are those included in the chosen database?
- Is this the only and/or best platform for this database? For example, Medline can be searched on the Ovid platform, which requires a subscription, and the PubMed platform, which is freely available. Which works best for the reviewer? Considerations include the reviewer's familiarity with the search interface, whether a platform links to available full-text literature, and whether the platform supports export to a citation management software. Definitions of platform and search interface appear in the next section. Reviewing the "About" section of a database's website can answer some of the questions above, as can consultation with a librarian.

Literature identified during the question formulation stage, or during preliminary searches, can help identify relevant databases. From an article citation found in a preliminary search, one can discover other databases in which the journal was indexed. For example, if a useful article is found in the *Journal of Pain and Symptom Management*, published by Elsevier, a visit to that journal's website reveals that it is indexed in multiple databases, including CINAHL, EMBASE, PubMed, Scopus, PyschInfo, and others, all of which may be considered for the IR. Exploring the "Methods" sections of published IRs on similar topics will also suggest possible databases.

3.3.2 Terminology

Database terminology can be confusing, especially because the words used may have different meanings in different disciplines. For the purposes of this chapter, the terms *platform, database, interface,* and *search engine* will be used as described below:

- A *platform* refers to the software used by a specific database provider. The platform does not always have the same name as the database. CINAHL is delivered on the EBSCO platform, while Medline is available on Ovid and ProQuest platforms.
- A *database* refers to an electronic, searchable collection of published materials, including some combination of journal articles, book chapters, reports, dissertations, and conference proceedings. Each database indexes a different set of resources and discloses information about those resources (titles, dates, publisher, etc.). Most databases are available through college, university, or hospital institutional subscriptions.
- A *search interface* refers to the search page and features that allow a user to search a database. Most search interfaces include basic and advanced search fields and a variety of limiters. Database search interfaces enable saving of search histories, which are needed to document the IR search process.
- The term *search engine* is used here to describe systems like Google, Google Scholar, Bing, and Yahoo, which enable users to search the World Wide Web. Unlike databases, search engines do not disclose exactly where and how they find their results; therefore, the search engine search process cannot be documented in the same way that the database search process can. The term *search engine* can also refer to resources beyond the popular examples shown here. Many libraries refer to their integrated search platform as a search engine, because it searches across multiple databases and includes the library catalog.

3.3.3 Nursing, Allied Health, and Medical Databases

Table 3.1 includes databases of literature in nursing, allied health, and medicine. Literature in these databases includes articles from scholarly journals published by multiple publishers, conference proceedings, and reports. All databases on this table, with the exception of PubMed, require access through subscription, and are most often available through a hospital; college; or university library. Depending upon the reviewer's institution, some databases may be available, but not all. For instance, CINAHL is the widely recognized and available through many hospitals, nursing schools, and some professional organizations including CINAHL access in its membership fee. Engaging a librarian in a discussion of which databases are available will support a decision about which should be included (Table 3.1).

Table 3.1 Databases for Nursing and Medical Literature

Database	Description	Publications	Platforms
CINAHL	Comprehensive database for nursing research and information. Indexes of peer-reviewed journals, books, conference proceedings, dissertations, and other publication types. Full text depends upon subscription level	Journal articles from multiple publishers; selected book chapters, conference proceedings, and standards of practice	EBSCOhost
Cochrane Library	A collection of databases that contains different types of evidence, including the Database of Systematic Reviews	Systematic reviews; Cochrane's content conforms to the Cochrane Handbook for Systematic Reviews of Interventions	CRD, EBSCO, Ovid, Wiley
EMBASE	Comprehensive index of biomedical literature, pharmacological information, and conference abstracts	Journal articles from multiple publishers; conference abstracts	Elsevier, Ovid
Joanna Briggs Institute	Summarized healthcare and nursing research and systematic review register and other tools to support evidence-based practice	Systematic reviews and research summaries	Ovid
Medline	From the US National Library of Medicine® (NLM), a comprehensive index of journal articles in life sciences with a concentration on biomedicine, indexed with NLM Medical Subject Headings (MESH®); included in PubMed	Journal articles from multiple publishers and some additional publications	PubMed, ProQuest, EBSCOhost, Web of Science, and Ovid
Proquest Nursing and Allied Health Database	Indexes of journal content from nursing literature and related disciplines. Claims more available full text than other databases	Journal articles from multiple publishers, dissertations, conference papers, and proceedings	Proquest

(continued)

Table 3.1 (continued)

Database	Description	Publications	Platforms
PubMed and PubMed Central	From the NLM, a comprehensive index of biomedical and life sciences journals, including nursing and allied health disciplines. PubMed contains all Medline content, plus additional citations; full-text articles are available through the PubMed Central interface	Journal articles from multiple publishers	National Center for Biotechnology Information
Scopus	Extensive database of scientific research, including health, life physical, and social sciences. Includes EMBASE index terms and citations	Journal articles and book chapters from multiple publishers	Elsevier
TRIP (Turning Research into Practice)	Indexes 500 journals with highest impact factors, all randomized controlled trials and systematic reviews included in PubMed, and all peer-reviewed articles included in PubMed Central	Journal articles from multiple publishers	TRIP
Web of Science	Extensive international multidisciplinary database which provides citation impact data.	Journal articles from multiple publishers, data sets	Clarivate Analytics

3.3.4 Interdisciplinary Databases

A reviewer may consider a question or questions from the perspective of economics, education, psychology, and sociology, among other disciplines. The librarian can be helpful in deciding whether databases in related disciplines should be included in the search strategy. As with nursing and medical databases, questions of availability must be considered. Table 3.2 illustrates examples of databases in related disciplines; this is not an exhaustive list, but it includes some major databases to consider. Like the databases in Table 3.1, databases in Table 3.2 may appear on more than one platform and will be accessible through institutional subscription, or possibly membership in a professional organization (Table 3.2).

3.4 Searching Systematically

Systematic database searching includes the methods described subsequently. Natural and controlled language, Boolean operators, and advanced search techniques are features of most databases, and when used together, they help to build an effective search.

Table 3.2 Examples of databases in related disciplines

Database	Description	Publications	Platforms
AgeLine (EBSCO)	Online resource for social gerontology research, focusing exclusively on issues of aging and the population of people aged 50 years and older	Journal articles, books, book chapters and reports	EBSCO
EconLit	Produced by the American Economic Association, covering economic literature.	Journal articles, book chapters, dissertations, working papers	EBSCO, Ovid, Proquest
Educational Resources Information Center: ERIC	Online library of education research and information, sponsored by the Institute of Education Sciences (IES) of the U.S. Department of Education	Education research, including journal articles and ERIC reports	EBSCO, Ovid, Proquest
E I Compendex	Indexes literature from 190 engineering disciplines, including numerous topics covering technology and health, e.g., wearable sensors, telemedicine, mobile applications	Journal articles, book chapters, dissertations, working papers	Elsevier
PsycInfo	APA's databases index research from publications in psychology, and the behavioral and social sciences. Includes interdisciplinary research.	Journal articles, book chapters, and dissertations	APA PsycNet, EBSOCOhost, Ovid, Proquest
Sociological Abstracts	Comprehensive research database for sociology and related disciplines including ethnic and racial studies, gender studies, marriage and family, psychology, religion, substance abuse, and violence	Journal articles, dissertations, books, conference papers, and proceedings	Proquest
SocIndex (EBSCO)	Sociology and related social sciences, ethnic and racial studies, gender studies, marriage and family, psychology, religion, substance abuse, violence.	Journal articles and book chapters from multiple publishers	EBSCO

3.4.1 Natural and Controlled Language

Keywords, or natural language search terms, can be identified by brainstorming about the review question and by reviewing article examples and search results found in preliminary searches. Searching with natural language terms will capture any results that include the term—whether the literature is "about" the topic or simply mentions it. Keyword searches usually return the greatest number of results, but not necessarily highest in relevance. Many databases use keyword or natural language searches as their default option.

Controlled vocabulary refers to a standardized predefined set of terms used by a database to describe and categorize articles or sources of information based on content. Subject terms may not be consistent across databases. Controlled vocabulary may also be called *controlled language subject headings* or *thesaurus terms*. MeSH (Medical Subject Headings), developed by the National Library of Medicine and assigned to articles in Medline, PubMed, CINAHL, Cochrane, and other databases, is an example of a controlled language. Most but not all databases use controlled language systems or thesaurus.

Reviewers are advised to begin with the familiar natural language, or keywords; find the most relevant search results, and within those, identify the controlled language, or subject terms, associated with those results. Controlled language searches may return fewer, but more relevant, results than natural language searches.

Both natural language and controlled language searches are important to include in the search strategy, because each method may yield different results. Figure 3.1 shows how a natural language example translates to controlled language terms in three different databases.

3.4.2   Combining Search Terms Using Boolean Logic

When natural and controlled language search terms have been identified through reading results from preliminary database searches, a revised search strategy can be formed. Whether using controlled or natural language, search terms are usually combined using the Boolean operators *AND*, *OR*, and *NOT*.

The operator *OR* will expand results and is usually used to combine similar terms. Often when typing a search term into a search box, a search string will appear

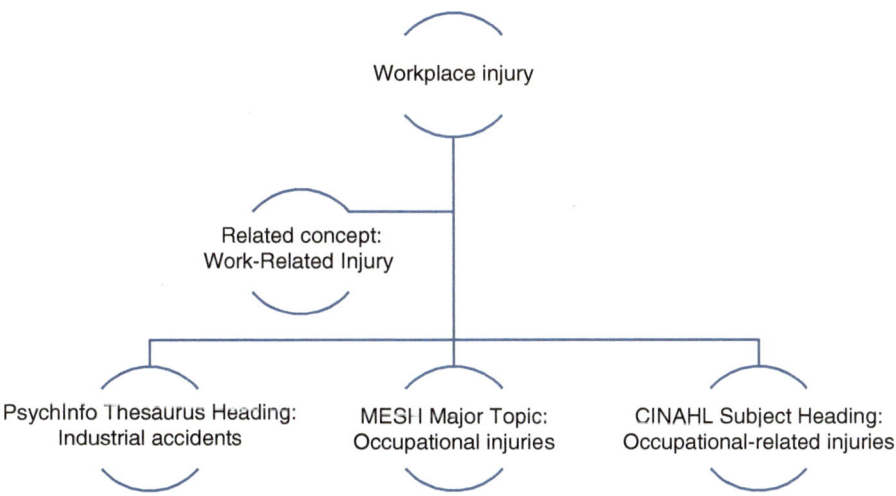

Fig. 3.1 From natural to controlled language (From: What to know about search queries EBSCO, ca. 2017)

using the *OR* operator, such as *teamwork OR collaboration OR mutual support*. This search will look for articles that include *any* of these search terms, or phrases. A library adage says *OR gets you more*.

The operator AND will identify articles which includes ALL of the search terms joined by *AND*: (*teamwork OR collaboration OR mutual support*) *AND* (*nursing students OR nursing education*) will only return articles that include references to search terms from both the first group and the second group. Using *AND* reduces the number of results.

When using *OR* and *AND*, it may be helpful to consider that applying these operators to a search yields counterintuitive results. In daily conversation, using *or* usually implies a limitation: "I will have pie *or* ice cream" means choosing only one. However, in Boolean searching, looking for a literature on *pie OR ice cream* will return literature on pie alone, ice cream alone, or on *both* concepts. Likewise, in conversation, using *and* implies addition: "I will have pie *and* ice cream" means choosing both. In Boolean searching, searching for *pie AND ice cream* will only return literature that address *both* pie and ice cream. Any literature on just pie, or just ice cream, will not appear.

The operator NOT excludes concepts. The search (*teamwork OR collaboration OR mutual support*) *AND* (*nursing students OR nursing education*) *NOT* (*hospital OR acute setting*) will return literature that includes teamwork and nursing students, but will not include references to hospitals. Such results may instead include literature about teamwork and nursing students in the community, or in the classroom. This is an approach to narrowing results by exclusion of search terms, rather than inclusion.

Boolean operators should be capitalized. Although some databases, including CINAHL, do not strictly require capitalized operators, there is a risk that using lower case for Boolean operators will result in those terms being searched as text, which will confuse search results. It is wiser to err on the side of caution (Cooper 1998).

3.4.3   Advanced Search Techniques

Advanced search techniques refine and focus search results and can be used to address exclusion and inclusion criteria. Each database interface provides a framework determining how limiters and search queries are represented, and while there are some similarities across databases, there are also variations. Understanding how each database uses advanced search techniques can support the return of relevant results. Some common techniques are shown subsequently:

• Common limiters found in many databases include *time frame, language, publication type, age of study participants*, and *geographic location*. The use of such limiters should align with the inclusion and exclusion criteria identified at question formulation stage, and if new limiters for criteria are determined during the search design process, they are documented and described in the review itself. An example can be seen in the Toronto and LaRocco (2019) IR, which identified a time period of 1994 through 2017, and justify their reason for beginning with 1994: because in that year, the first instance of a professional nursing organization publishing a statement on family presence appeared (Toronto and LaRocco 2019). This date was identified during preliminary searching.

- The *truncation* symbol replaces the ending, or final letters, of a search term, to capture all forms of that word. A common truncation symbol is the asterisk (∗), used by CINAHL, Embase, Medline, and PubMed. For example, the search term *cardio* ∗ will return instances of *cardiology* or *cardiovascular* and *cardiopulmonary*.
- *Parentheses* are used to group terms in a particular order, in the same way that parentheses in algebraic equations determine the order of operation. Boolean operators within parentheses indicate what combinations of terms to search and in what order. Search terms within parentheses are treated as a unit, and search terms without parentheses are searched from left to right. A search for *[(prostate cancer OR prostatic neoplasms) AND (screening OR assessment)]* will find articles about *prostate cancer OR prostatic neoplasms* (one unit) that also reference *screening OR assessment* (another unit). A search for the same terms without parentheses will not group terms as units, but combine them as directed by the Boolean operator, one term at a time.
- *Quotation marks* can be used around a phrase or concept of two or more words. Doing this instructs the database to search for the entire concept, rather than searching the terms separately. Searching the phrase "unpleasant symptoms" tells the database to search for exactly that phrase. Searching *unpleasant symptoms* without quotation marks will search for both terms, together or apart.
- The *wildcard* symbol replaces an unknown character, usually within a search term. A common wildcard symbol is the question mark (?), used in CINAHL, Embase, and Medline. For example, the search term *wom?n* will return instances of the terms *woman* or *women*; and *midwi?e* will return *midwife* and *midwive*.
- Proximity searching identifies search terms that appear near one another, but not necessarily next to each other. Searching for the search phrase *family presence* may return only results in that order of appearance. To find the literature where the concept of *family* and the concept of *presence* appear near one another (e.g., *family members who are present in the hospital*), proximity searches are useful and more precise than simply searching (famil∗ AND presen∗), which may produce results where those terms are not in relationship with one another. Proximity searches use designated letters combined with numbers to indicate the location of the terms. Databases use different proximity operators, which can usually be identified in the database help section.

3.5 Defining the Search Strategy

IRs are characteristically broad in nature. A review may explore how a theory has been applied to research or look for studies on the attitudes of a specific population toward a specific treatment, searching for literature on a concept or phenomenon rather than on the effectiveness of a clinical intervention. Using the review question(s) as a guide, key concepts are identified, related search terms are selected, and limiters identified, to focus the strategy. These steps require actively working within the selected databases. Westlake states: "The refinement of the question and the review of the literature is an iterative process that is recursive in nature, with the desired end point a fully refined … question with a matching review of the literature" (Westlake 2012, p. 245). As with all stages of the review, it is important to document preliminary searches, especially keeping track of any revisions made to the research question itself, or eligibility criteria.

Questions to consider in the early phase of searching: When does the topic or concept first appear in the database? Does the database include specific subject headings to support focused searching, or related terms to consider? Do preliminary findings suggest that the review question should be phrased differently or that the inclusion/exclusion criteria need reconsideration? The process of testing the search in this way supports further development of the search strategy.

Reviewers are encouraged to seek a balance between comprehensiveness (search recall or sensitivity) and relevance (search precision) (Levay and Craven 2018; National Institute for Health and Care Excellence 2014). The term recall is associated with how well a search captures all relevant literature, and the term precision is associated with how well a search avoids irrelevant results. The goal is to find as many relevant studies as possible, without being overwhelmed by results that are not useful. Clarifying concepts and search terms, and using limiters, can help.

3.5.1   Choosing Search Terms: Identifying Concepts

Concepts should be clearly defined in order to identify effective search terms (Evans 2007). Because many IRs deal with complex concepts or phenomena (such as dignity-conserving care actions in palliative care (Harstäde et al. 2018)), exploratory searches may be needed to uncover all relevant terms, after which synonyms for each concept can be identified. Below are two examples of integrative review questions and possible search strategies.

3.5.1.1 Identifying Concepts and Search Terms: Example 1
"What coping strategies are reported by family members of critically ill hospitalized patients?" (Rückholdt et al. 2019)

Concepts: Coping, family members, critically ill patients, hospital

Related terms and synonyms: coping, managing, tolerating; family members or family; critically ill patients, intensive care unit patients, critical care patient; hospital, acute setting, inpatient.

These terms can then be combined using some of the search methods mentioned above. Applying Boolean operators and truncation (∗) to these search terms would result in a search string such as this:

> (cop∗ OR manag∗ OR tolerat∗) AND (family member∗ OR family OR famil∗) AND (critically ill patient∗ OR intensive care unit patient∗ OR critical care patient∗) AND (hospital∗OR acute setting OR inpatient)

The above search string includes natural language terms—those that are identified by the reviewer, through brainstorming, and by reading about the subject. This search would yield results from which controlled language (or subject or thesaurus) terms could be identified. In CINAHL, some of the major subject headings associated with these search results include the following:

Critically ill patients; critical care; family coping; family role; caregivers—psychosocial factors; and stress management

Searching by major subject headings may return many of the same results as searching by natural language terms; nevertheless, a comprehensive search will include both methods. Any duplicate results can later be identified and removed.

3.5.1.2 Identifying Concepts and Search Terms: Example 2

"What are the transition-to-practice experiences of internationally educated nurses working in the United States?" (Ghazal et al. 2019, p. 5)

Concepts: Transition-to-practice experiences; internationally trained students; USA

Related terms and synonyms: transition to practice, internationally educated nurses, migrant nurses, foreign nurses, practice experience, United States, USA

A search string with Boolean operators and truncation (*) could look like this:

(internationally educated nurs* OR migrant nurs* OR foreign nurs*) AND (transition to practice OR practice experience OR practice) AND (United States OR USA)

CINAHL subject headings associated with search results include the following:

Foreign nurses, international nursing, transitional programs, practice patterns, workforce—United States

The examples described above illustrate possible search strategies and are not meant to suggest this is the only approach. Working with a librarian on this phase can support the reviewer's understanding of the search development process, which can seem ambiguous or not intuitive to the novice reviewer.

3.5.2 Document the Search Process

All search history (searches, search terms, results from those searches, and article citations) should be saved—even search results that may be excluded later. This information will be combined into a final reporting format, such as the PRISMA Flow Diagram (2015) or other type of search flow diagram.

Most colleges and universities provide subscription access to one or more citation managers, such as EndNote or RefWorks, so the reviewer will need to determine which software is available. Open-access citation management software like Zotero and Mendeley is freely available on the web and requires no institutional affiliation. When conducting the review with other authors, it is important to select a citation management software, which allows reviewers to share saved citations.

Articles saved to the reviewer's database user account can be exported to citation management software for the removal of duplicate articles from combined search results. Removing duplicates prior to screening for eligibility avoids unintended double counting of data, which can result in biased or incorrect review results

(Tramer et al. 1997). The number of duplicates removed will also be documented in the final reporting format.

Citation management software also offers integration with word processing software, facilitating creation of in-text citations from the reference list, and changing reference styles as needed suit publishing requirements. Tutorials describing exporting articles from databases, removal of duplicates, in-text citation support, and reference formatting can be found by a Google search of these subjects combined with the specific citation management software.

3.5.3   When Is the Database Search Process Complete?

Jewell, Fowler, and Foster include the following points made by Cooper and Valentine (Jewell et al. 2017):

- All databases likely to contain the highest number of citations have been searched.
- The search strategy has been modified by adding terms based on citations highly relevant to the topic.
- New searches return no new, unique, and relevant results.
- Author searches on the most prolific authors of the topic show no new citations.

Questions regarding the quality of the searches undertaken are raised by McGowan et al. McGowan et al. (2016, p. 42):

- The search concepts are clear, not too narrow or too broad.
- All spelling variants and synonyms have been searched, including abbreviations.
- Appropriate subject headings, or controlled language terms, have been identified and searched.
- Search limiters, filters, and Boolean operators have been used correctly.

3.6   Screening for Study Selection

Database search results, whether saved in citation management software or excel matrix, are next reviewed to determine which studies will be included in the review sample. The eligibility or inclusion/exclusion criteria guide the screening process. First, article titles are examined, and any duplicate or clearly irrelevant titles are removed. Next, reviewers look at the abstracts of any studies where there is any doubt of the relevance from the title—or, where it is impossible to judge relevance from the title alone. Citations with potentially relevant abstracts are identified as candidates for full-text screening. Citations determined to be irrelevant are excluded at this phase, and the number of citations excluded is documented. Once all potentially relevant studies have been identified, full-text articles for these citations are obtained and stored for further screening. Further literature may be excluded when the full text are screened, and these too should be documented (Whittemore and Knafl 2005). Table 3.3 illustrates how several published IRs applied inclusion and exclusion criteria to sample studies (Middlebrooks et al.

Table 3.3 Examples of documented inclusion and exclusion criteria

Author	Integrative review title	Inclusion and exclusion criteria applied during screening for eligibility
Middlebrooks, R., et al.	Effect of Evidence-Based Practice Programs on Individual Barriers of Workforce Nurses: An Integrative Review	During the eligibility phase, articles were excluded if the target sample consisted of only nurses in nonclinical roles, such as students, educators, or administrators. Articles that focused on specific guideline or protocol implementation without addressing the individual barriers to implementation of EBP were also excluded (Middlebrooks et al. 2016, pp. 399–400)
Vivieros, J., et al.	Meditation interventions among heart failure patients: An integrative review	Inclusion criteria for the integrative review were the following: (a) adult heart failure population (>18 years); (b) published in English; (c) identified as an empirical study, clinical trial, or randomized controlled trial; and (d) mindfulness or meditation as the intervention of study. Exclusion criteria included descriptive studies, abstracts, dissertations, and editorials. Additionally, trials that employed multicomponent interventions with exercise and meditation were excluded because the specific aspect of the intervention that contributed to any change could not be determined (Vivieros et al. 2019, p. 2)
Blakeman, J. R.	An integrative review of the theory of unpleasant symptoms	The inclusion criteria were purposefully broad, to provide a holistic picture of the Theory of Unpleasant Symptoms (TOUS) and its use in the research literature. Exclusion criteria included: (a) non-structured literature reviews, such as narrative reviews of the literature; (b) educational articles; (c) records related to concept and/or theory development; (d) dissertations; (e) records that only minimally used the TOUS where the TOUS was not used as a guide to the study; and (f) records applying a modified or hybrid version of the TOUS (Blakeman 2019, p 948).
Settecase-Wu, C.	Caring in the Nurse–Patient Relationship through the Caritas Lens: An Integrative Review	Inclusion criteria were English language, human subjects, qualitative and quantitative research, theoretical frameworks, and meta-analysis and integrative review studies. Criteria also included caring relationships within nursing. To ensure incorporation of recent literature, the limitation of "past 10 years" or the parameters 2008–2017 were imposed upon all searches. Studies referring to caring as a psychomotor action or implementation of tasks were eliminated. Other excluded works were reflective writings, editorials, informational pieces, inaccessible papers, and incomplete studies (findings only). All selected studies were anchored in the phenomena of caring (Settecase-Wu and Whetsel 2018, pp. 37–38)

2016; Vivieros et al. 2019; Blakeman 2019; Settecase-Wu and Whetsel 2018) (Table 3.3).

The process of searching databases, and screening results, is documented in the final review in narrative form and through a search flow diagram. The IR search flow diagram will be constructed after other search techniques and the gray literature have been investigated for additional studies. The flow diagram will include details of databases searched, records identified through database searching, number of records after duplicates removed, number of records screened, number of full-text records excluded (with reasons), and number of studies included in the final sample, as illustrated in the PRISMA Flow Diagram (2015). The next section addresses search techniques such as citation searching and non-database sources, sometimes referred to as gray literature.

3.7   Beyond Database Searching

The first part of the search focuses on developing well-crafted searches in databases engineered for discovery, and usually most of the records are peer-reviewed articles. The second part of the search involves processes to ensure that all relevant literature has been found by seeking different report formats, using resources other than databases, and utilizing other approaches for locating studies. Different report formats could be conference proceedings, dissertations, white papers, clinical trial registries, and more. Some of these formats are grouped together with the term gray literature, a term used for any reports that are not published in peer-reviewed journals or controlled by commercial publishers. These reports could be produced by a wide range of organizations—business or industry, government entities, academic institutions, or nonprofits—where publishing is not the primary activity. As these organizations are not focused on publishing, reports can be difficult to locate and require different search approaches. Added to that, it has been suggested that quality may be variable due to lack of peer review.

A good question to ask at this point would be—why is this necessary? The most important reason to consider searching beyond databases is minimize publication bias. This type of bias is defined as a situation that leads to a report not being published due to the nature of its results (Russell 2005). It is important to collect relevant literature to answer the IR research review question no matter the direction of the results in order to have the most comprehensive synthesis.

When designing a search in a database, the reviewer is dependent on the citation record to have certain concepts. However, reviewers do not always write abstracts including all the relevant concepts, and relevant thesaurus terms may not be added to the record. Some databases do not index all parts of a journal, leading to literature not being indexed in databases. Therefore, despite a reviewers' best efforts, relevant literature can be missed.

3.7.1   Gray Literature

Reports other than peer-reviewed literature can be difficult to find and can require knowledge about the field being studied to seek the most relevant sources to the proposed topic. This section will give a description of each type and provide examples of known sources.

3.7.2   Conference Proceedings

Many conferences create proceedings of posters, papers, and other events. Some conferences produce full reports for each event, while others provide abstracts only. Proceedings can be found by going directly to the conference website, seeking the printed proceedings, and searching a database that focuses on conference proceedings or a database that focuses on proceedings. The first step in searching proceedings would be to list relevant conferences to the review topic. From this list, determine which ones are available online or in print, or indexed in a database. More conferences are archiving proceedings online than ever before; however, not all conferences provide free access to their proceedings. Searching proceedings can mean browsing tables of contents online when/if other search options are not available. There are also conference databases that can quickly search across thousands of proceedings including databases that are interdisciplinary (Conference Proceedings Citation Index, COS Conference Papers Index, or Proceedings First), or databases that focus on one discipline like Northern Light from OVID, which covers biomedical conferences. Check with the library for availability as most of the databases are subscription based. Finally, some databases (CINAHL or ERIC) index conferences, but may not index the individual conference presentations. Once a conference report is found, it is important to check to see if it has been published, taking note that the title or first author might have been changed.

3.7.3   Dissertations/Theses

There are many benefits of including dissertations and theses for a comprehensive review. First, newer topics are often found in dissertations earlier than peer-reviewed publications. Second, dissertations are longer, providing more in-depth information about the literature, and tend to have more citations that could provide more information for the review. Finally, while the entire dissertation may be hundreds of pages long, the chapters on the study conducted may be shorter. The main difficulty in searching for dissertations is there is not one main place to search, but many sources. While Cumulative Index of Nursing and Allied Health Literature CINAHL (EBSCO) have index for some nursing dissertations, it will not index all, and many topics to be considered in IRs will cover a wide variety of fields (Table 3.4).

Table 3.4 Sources of dissertations

Resource	Link	Description
Networked Digital Library of Theses and Dissertations	search.ndltd.org/	Free
Open-Access Theses and Dissertations	oatd.org/	Free
ProQuest Dissertation/ Theses Global	www.proquest.com/ products-services/ dissertations/	Subscription based
Sigma Theta Tau/Virginia Henderson Repository	https://www.sigmarepository. org/	Free
WorldCat	www.worldcat.org/	Free catalog from libraries around the world: Tip: limit to dissertations

3.8 Additional Methods of Searching

After determining which types of literature to seek, it is time to select ways of searching for potential literature missed in the database searches.

3.8.1 Handsearching

Handsearching is one way to search for literature. In the past, searchers would physically gather 5–10 years of specific journal issues and flip through the pages looking for relevant literature. Today, this can be done electronically by searching table of contents of journals online. Other resources could also be searched through this process—conference proceedings, websites of relevant organizations, and more.

3.8.2 Citation/Related Article Searching

Reference searching also known as ancestry searching is looking at the reference lists of relevant resources—whether those are included in the review, related reviews, or important background articles to the topic. In addition, consider citation searching, looking for resources that have cited identified relevant resources. Both of these can be done most efficiently using one of the citation-tracking databases— Web of Science, Scopus, or Google Scholar. Out of these options, Scopus covers the most amount of journal titles while offering easy ways to collect and export citations (Mongeon and Paul-Hus 2016). These resources also offer related article searching, linking to other citations by the authors. Other resources also offer this feature, such as PubMed. It is important to use these features strategically, limiting how far away from the article these options are followed. Determine the process and time set aside for this type of search to limit the reach.

Table 3.5 Google example

Search	Exact search	Results
Google search without limiters	diabetes and (exercise or physical activity or walking)	41 million
Google search with limiters	diabetes and (exercise or physical activity or walking) and (file: .pdf or file: .org) and site: .edu or site: .org or site: .gov)	40

3.8.3 Subject Experts

Another way of finding literature not yet discovered through aforementioned meth-ods is to query subject experts and professional organizations. To start, create a description of the review and the literature to be included. Select potential authors, professional organizations, or other places based on the review search to date. Subject experts could be those who wrote the literature already identified to be included or those who have presented at conferences. Consider listing national and international organizations, similar to those considered when seeking conference papers, then determine if these organizations have a forum or listserv. Finally, post to the listserv forum or send the request to individual authors. Not only does this have the potential to yield literature that have been missed, it can also provide a networking opportunity.

3.8.4 Overall Gray Literature Resources

There are a few databases that can be searched for gray literature. Google Scholar is usually the first resource that comes to mind when thinking of this type of resource. Although Google Scholar does cover gray literature, Google can be more inclusive and, when searched strategically, provide a useful set of results (Bonato 2018). When searching Google, it is important to set parameters and a time limit as it could easily retrieve hundreds of thousands of results. Table 3.5 shows examples of a Google search with and without limiters. It is good to set a limit of how many results that will be reviewed, 100–200 to browse through maybe a reasonable number (Table 3.5).

3.9   Reporting the Search Strategy

Throughout the review process, it is important to carefully document the search conducted in each resource for reporting and updating needs. The most important thing to remember about the search report is that it needs to be presented in a way that each search could be reproducible or can at least be properly evaluated. This will require searches to be provided exactly as they were entered into the database. While saving searches within vendor sites (such as Ovid or Ebsco) is the most effi-cient way to update searches at a later date, copying and pasting the actual search

Table 3.6 Examples of reporting styles

Listing terms	Copying and pasting
Narrative:	Narrative:
The search consisted of the following terms: "exercise," "physical fitness," "physical activity" and "diabetes," "diabetics," "type 2 diabetes" Figure or table provided: none	The search consisted of keywords and thesaurus terms covering the concepts: exercise and diabetes. Figure or table provided: (AB (exercise or (physical n1 (activity or fitness)) or walk* or (resistance n1 train*) or (weight n1 lift*) or aerobic*) OR (MH "Exercise+") OR (MH "Resistance Training") OR (MH "Walking+") OR (MH "Aerobic Exercises+") OR (MH "Muscle Strengthening+")) AND (AB diabet* OR (MH "Diabetes Mellitus+")

Table 3.7 Documenting the searches/what to report

Type of search	Document
Database[a]	Database, vendor/interface, years covered by search, limits applied, copy and paste search (Cochrane Handbook)
Contacting authors	Describe who was contacted (such as first authors of included articles) and dates
Advertising for articles	Which listservs or forums were utilized
Browsing	List resources were browsed, years covered
Google	Copy and paste search; describe any parameters (such as looked at first 100 results)
Citing, Cited, Related search	Describe resources used, which articles were selected to start with in the search

[a]Includes any database—bibliographic database, trial registry, conference proceedings, and more

into a word document is also recommended. Searches should also be described narratively to provide additional details such as limiters that were applied or reasons behind decisions (Table 3.6).

In addition to providing the database searches, all other search methods need to be clearly described. Any limits applied, dates covered, and dates of the search are important to document so that the scope of the search is clearly described (Table 3.7).

3.9.1 Managing the Collected Data

Reviewers will need to describe the entire search process to the reader. After conducting a comprehensive search, all citations will be retrieved and labeled. This requires project management planning from the beginning of the review by developing protocols for each step and selecting tools to make the process more efficient. The first software to consider is citation manager to use in collecting and de-duplicating results. Next is a tool for sorting the records. While this can be done in the citation manager, other tools offer options to have more than one

Table 3.8 Types and examples of software to consider

Type of software	Name	Description
Bibliographic software All of these tools allow users to collect, manage, and cite resources	Endnote	Software to purchase and cost to update yearly; some sharing options
	RefWorks	Subscription online tool; easy to share and manage multiple projects; options to add citations from many source types
	Zotero	Free, online tool for managing citations; easy to share
Sorting	Rayyan ra	Free tool for sorting citations into include or exclude, or other custom labels; add files in multiple formats
	AbstractR	Free tool for labeling; works best with PubMed results
	SysRev	Free tool for sorting citations; works with PubMed; also add files from other databases; project management tools
Entire review process	Cadima	Free online tool for managing a review; form for describing scope of review; add citations from multiple sources; data extract tool; add team members
	Covidence	Free for the first review; add citations from multiple sources; data extract tool; creates PRISMA flowchart based on data
	DistillerSR	Subscription, online tool; provides many options for conducting all steps of the review; project management tools for working with teams

screener and ease in labeling articles included or excluded. Lastly, there is software designed to manage all of the review processes. Characteristics to consider are how well does the software interface with other software (such as spreadsheets), the time it takes to learn, and the cost. Potential tools to consider are listed in Table 3.8.

3.9.2 Screening, Selecting, and Sorting

When sorting the collected citations, there are three processes: screening by relevance, then selecting by full text, and finally sorting into studies. While these steps seem easy, this process can be challenging and time-consuming, and there are pitfalls to avoid. Each of these processes should be piloted before completing. In addition, it is important to document the process for reporting in the methods and results section of the review. The PRISMA flowchart (Pannucci and Wilkins 2010) is one way to display the flow of the records through the review process. It includes the number of records collected, screened, and selected. The reporting needs of each process are described in the sections further.

3.9.2.1 Screening for Relevancy

The first look at the collected citations is done by considering titles and/or abstracts. In this case, the process is to discard what is not relevant, that is, looking for reasons to kick out a citation, not looking to see that it matches all of the eligibility criteria. Abstracts are usually too brief or vague to find all of the required criteria, yet hopefully enough to see what is not relevant.

3.9.2.2 Selection

When selecting by full text, the report must have all of the required criteria. Have a plan in place for where the full text (usually pdf files) will be stored. It is also useful to have a naming structure when saving the files, such as first author followed as part of the title: Smith_PatientsWithDiabeticNeuropathy. While it is good to try and retrieve all of the full-text reports of potential literature, there may be some that cannot be found.

3.9.2.3 Sorting

The last part of this process is to sort the reports into studies. Most of the time one article is reporting on just one research project or study, while there are times when one study is described in more than one report, such as a dissertation and a journal article. Instead of counting those as two studies, it would be counted as one study, using both of the reports to collect data about the project. Sometimes one report is multiple studies, which should be treated separately.

3.9.3   Reporting Results of Screening and Selection

When reporting the results of screening and selection, this should be done both narratively and visually. There are different tools to help produce the PRISMA flowchart. First, PRISMA provides a template on its website (PRISMA Flow Diagram 2015) as a MS Word document or a pdf. One thing to note is that the PRISMA flowchart does not have to be exactly as shown in the template. The idea is to provide the information about the flow and the processes and the numbers, not that it must match the template exactly. Another option is to use a website like the PRISMA flowchart generator (Toronto Health Economics and Technology Assessment Collaborative n.d.) to create a flowchart which can be downloaded in a variety of formats including pdf, gif, and more. Lastly, Microsoft PowerPoint or other software helps in creating flowcharts or diagrams.

3.10   Conclusion

Many consider the search for an IR to be one phase of the review, but it is best to view it as an iterative process. It will require planning and can be greatly enhanced by collaborating with a librarian. There are standards to minimize publication bias and best practices to ensure efficiency. By selecting appropriate resources and software and setting realistic timelines, the search process will be less daunting and provide a comprehensive set of resources on which to base the review.

References

Blakeman JR (2019) An integrative review of the theory of unpleasant symptoms. J Adv Nurs 75(5):946–951. https://doi.org/10.1111/jan.13906

Bonato S (2018) Searching the grey literature. Rowman & Littlefield Publishers, Lanham, MA

Cooper HM (1982) Scientific guidelines for conducting integrative research reviews. Rev Educ Res 52(2):291–302. https://doi.org/10.3102/00346543052002291

Cooper HM (1998) Synthesizing research: a guide for literature reviews, 3rd edn. Sage Publications, Thousand Oaks

Cooper C, Booth A, Varley-Campbell J, Britten N, Garside R (2018) Defining the process to literature searching in systematic reviews: a literature review of guidance and supporting studies. BMC Med Res Methodol 18(1):8–3. https://doi.org/10.1186/s12874-018-0545-3

Coyne E, Rands H, Frommolt V, Kain V, Plugge M, Mitchell M (2018) Investigation of blended learning video resources to teach health students clinical skills: an integrative review. Nurse Educ Today 63:101–107. https://doi.org/10.1016/j.nedt.2018.01.021

Evans D (2007) Overview of methods. In: Webb C, Roe B (eds) Reviewing research evidence for nursing practice: systematic reviews. Blackwell Publishing, Oxford, pp 137–149

Fowler S (2017) Identifying the studies, Part 1: Database searching. In: Foster MJ, Jewell ST (eds) Assembling the pieces of a systematic review: a guide for librarians. Rowman & Littlefield, Lanham, MD, pp 67–84

Ganong LH (1987) Integrative reviews on nursing research. Res Nurs Health 10(1):1–11. https://doi.org/10.1002/nur.4770100103

Ghazal LV, Ma C, Djukic M, Squires A (2019) Transition-to-U.S. practice experiences of internationally educated nurses: an integrative review. West J Nurs Res 4:193945919860855. https://doi.org/10.1177/0193945919860855

Harstäde CW, Blomberg K, Benzein E, Östlund U (2018) Dignity-conserving care actions in palliative care: an integrative review of Swedish research. Scand J Caring Sci 32(1):8–23. https://doi.org/10.1111/scs.12433

Higgins JPT, Thomas J, Chandler J, Cumpston M, Li T, Page MJ, Welch VA (2019) Cochrane Handbook for Systematic Reviews of Interventions version 6.0 (updated July 2019). Cochrane. www.training.cochrane.org/handbook

Hopia H, Latvala E, Liimatainen L (2016) Reviewing the methodology of an integrative review. Scand J Caring Sci 30(4):662–669. https://doi.org/10.1111/scs.12327

Jewell ST, Fowler S, Foster MJ (2017) Identifying the studies, part 2: beyond database searching. In: Foster MJ, Jewell ST (eds) Assembling the pieces of a systematic review: a guide for librarians. Rowan & Littlefield, Lanham, MD, pp 85–97

Levay P, Craven J (2018) Introduction: where are we now? In: Craven J, Levay P (eds) Systematic searching: practical ideas for improving results. Facet Publishing, London

McGowan J, Sampson M, Salzwedel DM, Cogo E, Foerster V, Lefebvre C (2016) PRESS peer review of electronic search strategies: 2015 Guideline Statement. J Clin Epidemiol 75:40–46. https://doi.org/10.1016/j.jclinepi.2016.01.021

Middlebrooks R Jr, Carter-Templeton H, Mund AR (2016) Effect of evidence-based practice programs on individual barriers of workforce nurses: an integrative review. J Contin Educ Nurs 47(9):398–406. https://doi.org/10.3928/00220124-20160817-06

Moher D, Liberati A, Tetzlaff J, Altman DG (2009) Preferred reporting items for systematic reviews and meta-analyses: the PRISMA statement. PLoS Med 6(7):e1000097. https://doi.org/10.1371/journal.pmed.1000100

Mongeon P, Paul-Hus A (2016) The journal coverage of Web of Science and Scopus: a comparative analysis. Scientometrics 106(1):213–228. https://doi.org/10.1007/s11192-015-1765-5

National Institute for Health and Care Excellence. Developing NICE guidelines: the manual (2014). https://www.nice.org.uk/process/pmg20/resources/developing-nice-guidelines-the-manual-pdf-72286708700869 (p. 89–92). Accessed 17 Nov 2019

Pannucci CJ, Wilkins EG (2010) Identifying and avoiding bias in research. Plast Reconstr Surg 126(2):619–625. https://doi.org/10.1097/PRS.0b013e3181de24bc

PRISMA Flow Diagram (2015). http://www.prisma-statement.org/. Accessed 14 Oct 2019

Rückholdt M, Tofler GH, Randall S, Buckley T (2019) Coping by family members of critically ill hospitalised patients: an integrative review. Int J Nurs Stud 97:40–54. https://doi.org/10.1016/j.ijnurstu.2019.04.016

Russell CL (2005) An overview of the integrative research review. Prog Transplant 15(1):8–13. https://doi.org/10.1177/152692480501500102

Settecase-Wu C, Whetsel MV (2018) Caring in the nurse-patient relationship through the caritas lens: an integrative review. Cultura del Cuidado 15(2):34–66. https://doi.org/10.18041/1794-5232/cultrua.2018v15n2.5111

Soares CB, Komura Hoga LA, Peduzzi M, Sangaleti C, Yonekura T, Delage SD (2014) Integrative review: concepts and methods used in nursing. REV ESC ENFERMAGEM USP 48(2):329–339. https://doi.org/10.1590/S0080-623420140000200020

Tobiano G, Marshall A, Bucknall T, Chaboyer W (2015) Patient participation in nursing care on medical wards: an integrative review. Int J Nurs Stud 52(6):1107–1120. https://doi.org/10.1016/j.ijnurstu.2015.02.010

Toronto Health Economics and Technology Assessment Collaborative (Theta Collaborative) (n.d.) Citation 8. http://prisma.thetacollaborative.ca/. Accessed 17 Oct 2019

Toronto CE, LaRocco SA (2019) Family perception of and experience with family presence during cardiopulmonary resuscitation: an integrative review. J Clin Nurs (John Wiley & Sons Inc) 28(1):32–46. https://doi.org/10.1111/jocn.14649

Torraco RJ (2005) Writing integrative literature reviews: guidelines and examples. Hum Resour Dev Rev 4(3):356–367. https://doi.org/10.1177/1534484305278283

Torraco RJ (2016) Writing integrative literature reviews: using the past and present to explore the future. Hum Resour Dev Rev 15(4):404–428. https://doi.org/10.1177/1534484316671606

Tramer MR, Reynolds DJ, Moore RA, McQuay HJ (1997) Impact of covert duplicate publication on meta-analysis: a case study. BMJ 315(7109):635–640. https://doi.org/10.1136/bmj.315.7109.635

Vivieros J, Chamberlain B, O'Hare A, Sethares KA (2019) Meditation interventions among heart failure patients: an integrative review. Eur J Cardiovasc Nurs 18(8):720–728. https://doi.org/10.1177/1474515119863181

Westlake C (2012) Practical tips for literature synthesis. Clin Nurse Spec 26(5):244–249. https://doi.org/10.1097/NUR.0b013e318263d766

Whittemore R (2007) Rigour in integrative reviews. In: Webb C, Roe B (eds) Reviewing research evidence for nursing practice: systematic reviews. Blackwell Publishing, Oxford, pp 149–156

Whittemore R, Knafl K (2005) The integrative review: updated methodology. J Adv Nurs 52(5):546–553. https://doi.org/10.1111/j.1365-2648.2005.03621.x

Quality Appraisal

4

Ruth Remington

Contents

4.1   Applying Inclusion Criteria.. 45
4.2   Identifying Methodological Rigor.. 46
4.3   Sources of Bias.. 46
4.4   Validity.. 48
4.5   Critical Appraisal Tools.. 48
    4.5.1   Design Specific Versus Generic... 50
    4.5.2   Appraisal of Theoretical Literature.. 51
    4.5.3   Appraisal of Gray Literature... 51
4.6   Applicability of Results.. 52
    4.6.1   Reporting Guideline Versus Appraisal Tool.. 53
4.7   Conclusion.. 53
References... 53

4.1   Applying Inclusion Criteria

Critical appraisal of quality has been described as a systematic examination of literature to evaluate its reliability, value, and relevance in a particular context (Mhaskar et al. 2009). It is important to note that published studies can be of varying quality. Including poor quality studies in the review may distort the synthesis, whereas excluding studies of poor quality may bias the synthesis (Evans 2007).

Therefore, the inclusion and exclusion criteria should identify whether inferior studies will be included or excluded after the appraisal process. Some suggest that all studies should be considered in the review, despite low-quality ratings to allow for more diversity among the sample, whereas others suggest that synthesizing studies of high quality with those of lesser quality may lead to inaccurate conclusions

R. Remington (✉)
Department of Nursing, Framingham State University, Framingham, MA, USA

© Springer Nature Switzerland AG 2020   45
C. E. Toronto, R. Remington (eds.), *A Step-by-Step Guide to Conducting an Integrative Review*, https://doi.org/10.1007/978-3-030-37504-1_4

(Mi 2017). Whether or not to synthesize all relevant works in the integrative review (IR) is one of several important decisions that need to be made at this stage of the IR; however, it is essential that all evidence be assessed for quality before inclusion in the IR. The relevance of the literature to the review question should guide the decision to include or exclude literature on the basis of quality. Keeping the review question at the forefront as each decision is made will help to keep the process on track and help to avoid unintended digression.

4.2   Identifying Methodological Rigor

Integrative reviews should be conducted with as much rigor as in the studies they summarize (Hawker et al. 2002). Since 1980, four seminal papers have called for evaluation of the quality of data included in IRs (Jackson 1980; Ganong 1987; Cooper 1989; Whittemore 2005), yet IRs continue to be published without addressing this important step in the process (Toronto et al. 2018). Reviewers should make judgments about the methodological strengths and weaknesses of all included studies before making inferences about the phenomenon of interest (Jackson 1980), in order to achieve rigor in the IR.

Methodological rigor is associated with the quality of the research. The quality of studies has been described as the extent to which the study uses measures to minimize bias in the design, conduct, and analysis of the research. Bias is anything that systematically or predictably distorts the results of a study in a way that is different from the truth. The presence of bias influences the believability or trustworthiness of the results (Salmond 2012). In addition to bias, other aspects of studies are often included in the assessment of quality, such as statistical power, ethical approval (Mi 2017; Sanderson et al. 2007; Harder et al. 2014), and the agreement between the review question and the method used (Melnyk and Fineout-Overholt 2014).

4.3   Sources of Bias

Bias can occur at any stage of the research. Identifying the risk of bias begins by looking at each study for potential sources of bias. The method of assessing the risk of bias should be transparent and reproducible. This focus on bias or believability of findings is referred to as internal validity. Common types of bias in studies include selection, measurement, attrition, and performance bias and are described in Table 4.1.

The quantitative understanding of bias is not well matched with qualitative research paradigm. In quantitative research, bias affects the reliability and validity of the findings. The qualitative concept of rigor is known as trustworthiness which is composed of four components: transferability, credibility, confirmability, and dependability (Williams et al. 2019). Although these criteria are different, they mirror the concerns of reliability and validity in quantitative research (Garside 2014) and are described in Table 4.2.

Table 4.1 Potential sources of bias

Type	Description	Example	Strategies to Minimize
Selection	Problems in allocating study participants to groups in a way that results in systematic differences between study groups	In a study of women and heart disease, one group had more health conscious, thinner, physically active women with better access to health care	Minimized by randomization or concealment of allocation from data collectors
Measurement	Inconsistency in measuring study outcomes resulting in a difference between the measured variable and its actual value	Survey interviewer in a diet study was poorly trained and neglected to collect complete intake for one of the study groups	Minimized by training research personnel and using measurement instruments with high precision
Attrition	Participants who drop out and are lost to follow up differ systematically from those who complete the study	In a weight loss study, the heaviest participants dropped out	Intention-to-treat analysis or description of withdrawals in report
Performance	One group of study participants receives more attention or care than another study group resulting in systematic differences between study groups	Participants in one group learn that they are receiving the new treatment and may experience placebo effects	Minimized by blinding and/or use of a standardized protocol

Table 4.2 Concepts of trustworthiness in qualitative research

Criterion	Description	Strategies
Transferability	Ability to transfer conceptual findings to other settings	Thick description of the participants and context
Credibility	Research account is believable and appropriate	Peer debriefing, independent analysis by more than one researcher, verbatim quotes
Dependability	Methods and decisions logical, traceable, and clearly documented	Peer review, debriefing, audit trails, triangulation of methods
Confirmability	Extent to which findings are grounded in the data	Triangulation, reflexivity, assess effect of researcher on the research process

Publication bias is a common problem that occurs when publication is associated with the significance of the results. It has been estimated that nearly 50% of completed clinical trials are not published (Paez 2017). Journals often fail to publish studies that are not significant on the basis of the direction or strength of the outcome of interest. Similarly, authors may be reluctant to devote the time to prepare and submit a manuscript with negative results that they believe may not be publishable. Studies with negative or nonsignificant results are less likely to be published than those with positive results, making published works systematically different from unpublished, completed studies (Song et al. 2013). Additionally, gray literature (theses, dissertations, conference papers, government reports, policy papers, etc.)

is not included in computerized bibliographic databases making potentially valuable data difficult to find, resulting in publication bias (Aromataris and Munn 2017; Polkki et al. 2013).

4.4 Validity

Validity refers to how closely the results of the study approximate the truth. Validity is demonstrated when results of the study are obtained using proper scientific methods. Bias can compromise the validity of individual study results and lead to a biased IR, potentially resulting in the over- or underestimation of the effect (Sanderson et al. 2007; Harder et al. 2014). External validity, or the degree to which the study results are generalizable or applicable to one's population of interest, is considered by some to be of equal importance in critical appraisal (Harder et al. 2014). It has been suggested by others that the appraisal should focus on internal validity (risk of bias, believability), as the applicability of the results (external validity) may depend on how the results are to be used, and if there is significant bias present, the results cannot be trustworthy (Higgins et al. 2011).

4.5 Critical Appraisal Tools

There is no consensus on the best way to appraise study quality; however, there is overwhelming agreement that any included studies and other evidence in an integrative review should be critically appraised (Katrak et al. 2004). Selecting the most appropriate critical appraisal tool to evaluate literature for the IR can be challenging for the novice as well as for the experienced reviewer (Buccheri and Sharifi 2017). The use of different appraisal tools can lead to different conclusions about the quality when applied to the same study.

There is much variability in the design and complexity of available critical appraisal tools. The items in appraisal tools are usually either open questions, closed questions, or statements. Open-ended questions and statements provide for a richer examination of data; however, closed questions are easier to analyze, score, and/or rank the studies (Crowe and Sheppard 2011). Since there has been no gold standard tool identified for determining quality (Whittemore 2005), many appraisal tools have been developed. More than 100 appraisal tools have been identified to appraise methodological quality of primary research (Sanderson et al. 2007; Katrak et al. 2004; Quigley et al. 2019). Nine critical appraisal tools were found to be commonly used in nursing, four of which can be used to appraise multiple study designs (Buccheri and Sharifi 2017) and are described in Table 4.3.

To further ensure accuracy and minimize bias in the critical appraisal process, it is preferable to have two reviewers independently review all literature for quality and relevance (Whittemore 2007). When completed, both reviewers should

Table 4.3 Selected design specific critical appraisal tools used in nursing

	Systematic review	Randomized controlled trial	Cohort study	Case-controlled study	Qualitative study	
Critical Appraisal Skills Program (CASP)	X	X	X	X	X	https://casp-uk.net/casp-tools-checklists/
Joanna Briggs Institute (JBI)	X	X	X	X	X	https://joannabriggs.org/critical_appraisal_tools
Johns Hopkins research evidence appraisal tool	X	X	X		X	https://www.hopkinsmedicine.org/eviden ce-based-practice/ijhn_2017_ebp.html
Rapid critical appraisal checklists	X	X	X	X	X	Melnyk & Fineout-Overholt. Evidence-based practice in nursing and healthcare. Philadelphia: Wolters Kluwer, 2015

compare their appraisals and discuss any areas of disagreement. If not resolved by discussion, a third reviewer should be consulted for adjudication (Aromataris and Munn 2017). The report of the review should clearly indicate how each article was appraised, what criteria were used to determine quality, and what the results of the appraisal were. Additionally, the report should identify whether any works were excluded based on the quality appraisal.

An example of the method proposed to exclude literature on the basis of relevance and quality is found in the IR of how nurse educators prepare nursing students for the emotional challenges of practice, conducted by Dwyer and Revell (2015, p. 9). The authors clearly described how the literature was evaluated for rigor and relevance.

Due to the inclusion of both empirical and nonempirical literature, the data were evaluated using a 2-point scale (2 = *high* or 1 = *low*) for two categories: data rigor and data relevance (Whittemore 2005). Data rigor was evaluated using a modified data appraisal protocol designed to assess methodological rigor of empirical studies (Hawker et al. 2002). Nonempirical articles were scored as not applicable. Data relevance was reviewed in reference to the ability of the data to contribute to the identified guiding questions. No article was excluded following the data evaluation process (p. 9).

4.5.1 Design Specific Versus Generic

Most appraisal tools are study design specific. Criteria relevant to each study design are evaluated. For example, blinding and randomization are critical areas for evaluation of a randomized controlled trial, but not relevant to a cohort or qualitative study. Therefore, the use of two or more critical appraisal tools may be necessary for completing a review containing multiple study designs. This may make it difficult to directly compare data from studies that use different designs and synthesize into a logical whole (Crowe and Sheppard 2011). Some authors recommend against the use of appraisal tools that produce composite scores as many give equal weight to each domain assessed, despite the relative value of that domain (Quigley et al. 2019). For example, if the appraisal tool rates the title with the same weight as the appropriateness of the design, it may obscure the impact of an inadequate design in the composite score.

Many appraisal tools are checklists addressing the presence or absence of essential items using a "yes," "no," or "not applicable" response format. Some provide a summary rating of overall quality. This response format facilitates rapid appraisal (Quigley et al. 2019). Some appraisal tools provide a score for each item that is totaled to produce a summary score that can be used to rank studies. The problem with a summary score is that a total score may be acceptable, but it may hide a serious flaw in the study if most of the items scored high. Other appraisal tools use a component score in which each component of the tool is compared across studies (Crowe and Sheppard 2011).

Another approach is to use a generic tool, evaluating criteria that could be applied to all included studies. In a review of critical appraisal tools ($n = 44$), six claimed to be applicable to all research designs (Crowe and Sheppard 2011). One of these has been developed in nursing and is presented with a comprehensive description the method used in its development (Hawker et al. 2002). Generic critical appraisal tools have been criticized because they are not specific to study design and related potential biases (Quigley et al. 2019). However, this type of critical appraisal tool does not place study design in a hierarchy so that the appraisal of studies of qualitative, quantitative, and mixed methods designs is based on the quality of each study within its own methodological domain (Pace et al. 2012). For example, all cohort studies within a review that use a generic appraisal tool are evaluated as to how well they addressed the potential for bias in the design of a cohort study, not according to a hierarchy of evidence based on study design. Generic appraisal tools may facilitate the synthesis of research of multiple designs that can increase the richness of the conclusions.

Methodological rigor is often judged by the hierarchy of evidence, basing the quality appraisal on the study design, not on other relevant aspects of quality. While it is true that studies conducted using methods higher in the hierarchy such as the randomized controlled trial are likely to be less prone to bias, the hierarchy alone does not address validity, reliability, and objectivity (Coryn 2007). A badly designed randomized clinical trial may be of lesser quality, even though the design is toward the top of the hierarchy. Moreover, many nursing questions are best answered by study designs lower in the hierarchy. For example, observational studies generally have less restrictive criteria and greater risk for bias, but better reflect the population that nursing serves (Salmond 2012).

4.5.2   Appraisal of Theoretical Literature

The option to include theoretical articles in the review distinguishes the IR from the systematic review. Theoretical articles examine existing literature and theories to advance the theoretical foundations of the discipline and cannot be appraised using tools similar to those used to appraise research literature focusing on reliability and study design (Campbell et al. 2014). The author of a theoretical article presents a new theory, analyzes an existing theory, or elaborates a theoretical position. These articles do not contain existing empirical information unless it advances the theoretical issue (American Psychological Association 2010).

Walker and Avant (2019) propose a six-step procedure for analyzing theory. In appraising the theoretical literature, the authors recommend to examine or analyze the following:

1. The origins, or the purpose for the initial development of the theory its assumptions, and any evidence that supports or refutes it
2. The meaning of the theory, its concepts and statements, their definitions and use, and how they relate to each other
3. The logical adequacy, or structure of the theory to identify whether the conclusions and the evidence they are based on make sense. The ability of the theory to make accurate predictions is examined
4. The usefulness of the theory or how helpful it is in understanding or predicting outcomes and the ability of the theory to generate research studies
5. Generalizability or transferability is the degree to which research findings can be applied to persons similar to those who were actually studied. It describes how broad the theory is and how well it can be applied to explain or predict phenomena. Parsimony describes how well complex phenomena are explained simply or briefly, while being complete in its explanation.
6. Testability refers to how well the theory can be supported by empirical data.

4.5.3   Appraisal of Gray Literature

Another decision that should be made early in the IR process is whether to include gray literature in the sample. Gray literature refers to papers that have not been published in commercial or academic journals and may include theses, dissertations, white papers, government, business, or academic documents that are protected by intellectual property rights but have not been distributed or indexed by commercial publishers or published in a traditional venue (Salmond 2012; Aromataris and Munn 2017). If the phenomenon of interest is well defined in the literature and there is a large volume of peer-reviewed, high-quality, published literature, gray literature may not add to the review. However, if the volume and quality of published literature are insufficient to address the review question, then gray literature may provide a rich source of data and context to the review (Benzies et al. 2006).

Evaluating the quality of gray literature can be a complex process. Not all gray literature is subjected to a peer-reviewed process (Adams et al. 2016b). Gray literature can range from opinion-driven, biased literature, to high-quality unpublished research (Benzies et al. 2006). Theses and dissertations are generally rigorously reviewed and likely to appraise as high quality. Similarly, conference abstracts and proceedings are typically peer reviewed by the organization presenting the conference, before they are accepted. Nearly half of conference presentations go on to be published, making conference proceedings another source of research to explore (Paez 2017). Dissertations and conference proceedings, if appraised and found to be relevant, may be good choices of gray literature to include in an IR if needed to supplement published data.

Gray literature also has the potential to reduce the influence of publication bias (Adams et al. 2016a); however, it is important that it be critically appraised before inclusion in the IR, as the quality of gray literature is variable. Unpublished research studies, such as dissertations, should be appraised using the appropriate critical appraisal tool as would be used for a published study. Other textual papers should be assessed for aspects such as accuracy, objectivity, authority, evidence, and significance. Examples of critical appraisal tools that can be used for gray literature include Joanna Briggs Institute NOTARI checklist (https://joannabriggs.org/critical_appraisal_tools) and the Johns Hopkins Non-Research Evidence Appraisal Tool (https://www.hopkinsmedicine.org/evidence-based-practice/_docs/appendix_f_non-research_evidence_appraisal_tool.pdf) or the AACODS Checklist (https://canberra.libguides.com/c.php?g=599348&p=4148869). When including gray literature, the reviewer should be aware that it may not be possible for others to replicate the search, as can be done with electronic databases (Adams et al. 2016b). Therefore, it is essential to provide a clear and comprehensive discussion of how the gray literature was identified to provide transparency in search methods.

4.6   Applicability of Results

While there is considerable variability in the construction of critical appraisal tools, most include items or description of the following:

- Preamble (title, text abstract)
- Introduction
- Design
- Sampling
- Data collection
- Ethical matters
- Results
- Discussion
- Relevance to the guiding question(s)

Notation of the results of the appraisal of each study should be entered into the matrix to support the credibility of the data analysis and findings of the review.

4.6.1 Reporting Guideline Versus Appraisal Tool

The quality of a research report cannot be assumed to reveal the quality of the research. Reporting guidelines such as the Preferred Reporting Items for Systematic Reviews and Meta- Analyses (PRISMA) is used to minimize bias in the reporting of the final review, focusing on how the final review should be written. The focus is how the review as a whole is reported, rather than how each included piece of literature is appraised (Crowe and Sheppard 2011).

The PRISMA guideline was developed to increase quality and transparency in reporting of the systematic review by describing a minimum set of characteristics to report in a systematic review. IRs should also exhibit transparency in reporting by following an established guideline. As further review-specific reporting guidelines are developed such at the PRISMA Extension for Scoping Reviews (PRISMA-ScR), closer alignment to the IR method will occur (Tricco et al. 2018).

4.7 Conclusion

Critical appraisal of literature included in the IR is essential to the rigor of the review. Many critical appraisal tools are available, but none has been universally accepted. Choosing the best tool for the review is a challenge for the writer. Keeping the review purpose and questions in the forefront will guide the appraisal process. Transparency and consistency in the description of the method(s) used to appraise the included literature will enhance the rigor of the IR.

References

Adams J, Hillier-Brown FC, Moore HJ, Lake AA, Araujo Soares V, White M et al (2016a) Searching and synthesizing 'grey literature' and 'grey information' in public health: critical reflections on three case studies. Syst Rev 5. https://doi.org/10.1186/s13643-016-0337-y

Adams RJ, Smart P, Huff AS (2016b) Shades of Grey: guidelines for working with the grey literature in systematic reviews for management and organizational studies. Int J Manag Rev 19:432–454. https://doi.org/10.1111/ijmr.12102

American Psychological Association (2010) Publication manual of the American Psychological Association, 6th edn. American Psychological Association, Washington, DC

Aromataris E, Munn Z (eds) (2017) Joanna Briggs Institute Reviewer's Manual. The Joanna Briggs Institute. https://reviewersmanual.joannabriggs.org/

Benzies KM, Shahirose P, Hayden A, Serrett K (2006) State of the evidence reviews: advantages and challenges of including grey literature. Worldviews Evid-Based Nurs 3:55–61

Buccheri RK, Sharifi C (2017) Critical appraisal tools and reporting guidelines for evidence-based practice. Worldviews Evid-Based Nurs 14:463–472. https://doi.org/10.1111/wvn.12258

Campbell M, Egan M, Lorenc T, Bond L, Popham F, Fenton C et al (2014) Considering methodological options for reviews of theory: illustrated by a review of theories. Syst Rev 3:114–125. https://doi.org/10.1186/2046-4053-3-114

Cooper HM (1989) Integrating research: a guide for literature reviews, 2nd edn. Sage, Newbury Park, CA

Coryn CLS (2007) The holy trinity of methodological rigor: a skeptical view. J Multi Discip Eval 4:26–31

Crowe M, Sheppard L (2011) A review of critical appraisal tools show they lack rigor: alternative tool structure is proposed. J Clin Epidemiol 64:80–89. https://doi.org/10.1016/j.jclinepi.2010.02.008

Dwyer PA, Revell SMH (2015) Preparing students for the emotional challenges of nursing: an integrative review. J Nurs Educ 54:7–12. https://doi.org/10.3928/01484834-20141224-06

Evans D (2007) Overview of methods. In: Webb C, Roe B (eds) Reviewing research evidence for nursing practice: in systematic reviews. Blackwell Publishing, Malden, MA, pp 137–148

Ganong LH (1987) Integrative reviews of nursing research. Res Nurs Health 10:1–11

Garside R (2014) Should we appraise the quality of qualitative research reports for systematic reviews, and if so, how? Innovation 27:67–79. https://doi.org/10.1080/13511610.2013.777270

Harder T, Takla A, Rehfuess E, Sanchez-Vivar A, Matysiak-Klose D, Eckmanns T et al (2014) Evidence-based decision-making in infectious diseases epidemiology, prevention and control: matching research questions to study designs and quality appraisal tools. BMC Med Res Methodol 14:69. https://doi.org/10.1186/1471-2288-14-69

Hawker S, Payne S, Kerr C, Hardey M, Powell J (2002) Appraising the evidence: reviewing disparate data systematically. Qual Health Res 12:1284–1299. https://doi.org/10.1177/104973230223851

Higgins JPT, Altman DG, Gotzsche PC, Juni P, Moher D, Oxman AD et al (2011) The Cochrane Collaboration's tool for assessing risk of bias in randomized trials. BMJ 343:d5928. https://doi.org/10.1136/bmj.d5928

Jackson GB (1980) Methods for integrative reviews. Rev Educ Res 50:438–460

Katrak P, Bialocerkowski AE, Massy-Westropp N, Kumar VS, Grimmer KA (2004) A systematic review of the content of critical appraisal tools. BMC Med Res Methodol 4. https://doi.org/10.1186/1471-2288-4-22

Melnyk BM, Fineout-Overholt E (2014) Evidence-based practice in nursing & healthcare, 3rd edn. Wolters Kluwer, Philadelphia

Mhaskar R, Emmanuel P, Nishra S, Patel S, Eknath N, Kumar A (2009) Critical appraisal skills are essential to informed decision-making. Indian J Sex Transm Dis AIDS 30:112–119. https://doi.org/10.4103/2589-0557.62770

Mi M (2017) Evaluating study selection and critical appraisal. In: Foster MJ, Jewell ST (eds) Assembling the pieces of a systematic review: a guide for librarians. Rowman & Littlefield, Lanham, MD, pp 125–145

Pace R, Pluye P, Gartlett G, Macaulay AC, Salsberg J, Jagosh J et al (2012) Testing the reliability and efficiency of the pilot Mixed Methods Appraisal Tool (MMAT) for systematic mixed studies review. Int J Nur Stud 49:47–53. https://doi.org/10.1016/j.ijnurstu.2011.07.002

Paez A (2017) Gray literature: an important resource in systematic reviews. J Evid Based Med 10:233–240. https://doi.org/10.1111/jebm.12265

Polkki T, Kanste O, Kaariainen M, Elo S, Kyngas H (2013) The methodological quality of systematic reviews published in high-impact nursing journals: a review of the literature. J Clin Nurs 23:315–332. https://doi.org/10.1111/jocn.12132

Quigley JM, Thompson JC, Halfpenny NJ, Scott DA (2019) Critical appraisal of nonrandomized studies-a review of recommended and commonly used tools. J Eval Clin Pract 25:44–52. https://doi.org/10.1111/jep.12889

Salmond SW (2012) Critical appraisal. In: Holly C, Salmond SW, Saimbert MK (eds) In comprehensive systematic review for advanced nursing practice. Springer, New York, pp 147–162

Sanderson S, Tatt ID, Higgins JPT (2007) Tools for assessing quality and susceptibility to bias in observational studies in epidemiology: a systematic review and annotated bibliography. Int J Epidemol 36:666–676. https://doi.org/10.1093/ije/dym018

Song F, Hooper L, Loke YK (2013) Publication bias: what is it? How do we measure it? How do we avoid it? Open Access J Clin Trials 3:71–81. https://doi.org/10.2147/OAJCT.S34419

Toronto CE, Quinn B, Remington R, (2018) Characteristics of reviews published in nursing literature: a methodological review. ANS Adv Nurs Sci 41(1):30–40. https://doi.org/10.1097/ANS.0000000000000180

Tricco AC, Lillie E, Zarin W, O'Brien KK, Colquhoun H, Levac D et al (2018) PRISMA extension for scoping reviews (PRISMA-ScR): checklist and explanation. Ann Intern Med 169:467–473. https://doi.org/10.7326/M18-0850

Walker LO, Avant KC (2019) Strategies for theory construction in nursing, 6th edn. Pearson, New York

Whittemore R (2005) Combining evidence in nursing research: methods and implications. Nurs Res 54:56–62

Whittemore R (2007) Rigour in integrative reviews. In: Webb C, Roe B (eds) Reviewing research evidence for nursing practice: in systematic reviews. Blackwell Publishing, Malden, MA, pp 149–156

Williams V, Boylan A, Nunan D (2019) Critical appraisal of qualitative research: necessity, partialities and the issue of bias. BMJ Evid Based Med. https://doi.org/10.1136/bmjebm-2018-111132

Analysis and Synthesis

5

Patricia A. Dwyer

Contents

5.1   Data Analysis and Synthesis... 57
5.2   Strategies for Data Analysis... 58
     5.2.1   Creating a Data Matrix... 58
     5.2.2   Data Analysis Methods... 60
5.3   Descriptive Results... 68
5.4   Synthesis.. 68
References.. 69

5.1   Data Analysis and Synthesis

Data analysis and synthesis are a challenging stage of the integrative review process. The description of explicit approaches to guide reviewers through the data analysis stage of an integrative review (IR) is underdeveloped (Whittemore and Knafl 2005). Furthermore, when reviewers look to published IRs for assistance, they often find the data analysis stage is only briefly and/or superficial described (Hopia et al. 2016).

So where does one begin? An important starting point is to understand that the primary goal of an IR is to create a better understanding of a topic through synthesis of diverse sources (Torraco 2016). Torraco defines synthesis as a creative process that generates a new model, conceptual framework, or other unique conception informed by the author's intimate knowledge of the topic (2005, p. 362). The results of the IR should not be a "data dump" (Torraco 2005, p. 362) or a series of summaries of each piece of literature (laundry listing). Instead, the goal is to make a new whole by

P. A. Dwyer (✉)
Boston Children's Hospital, Waltham, MA, USA

© Springer Nature Switzerland AG 2020   57
C. E. Toronto, R. Remington (eds.), *A Step-by-Step Guide to Conducting an Integrative Review*, https://doi.org/10.1007/978-3-030-37504-1_5

integrating smaller pieces of data (evidence) from different literature sources in the sample (Booth 2012).

Blondy et al. (2016) argue that true synthesis results in new meaning and knowledge transformation. Yet even when reviewers understand that synthesis is the desired outcome, they still struggle with how to get there. It is often helpful to conceptualize the data analysis stage of an IR as a vital process to help achieve synthesis. By using rigorous methods of data analysis, a reviewer will be able to recast, combine, reorganize, and integrate concepts across a body of literature to create new knowledge about their topic of interest (Torraco 2016).

5.2   Strategies for Data Analysis

5.2.1   Creating a Data Matrix

Data analysis of a body or sample of literature often requires the reviewer to first deconstruct each literature source into its most basic elements (Torraco 2005). One of the essential first steps in the data analysis stage is the creation of a review matrix (Garrard 2017). The review matrix provides a structured document to use during analysis and supports the writing of a narrative synthesis (Garrard 2017). A review matrix is a table that includes both rows and columns and is used to abstract data from published research or scholarly articles. The table can be created in a word processing document (Microsoft Word, Google Docs), an Excel spreadsheet, or a commercial literature review software program. The left side of the table includes a row for each literature source included in the sample. Across the top of the table is a series of columns that outline the key information to abstract from each source. There are no set of column topics; however, it is strongly recommended that the first three columns record fundamental information from the published source (Garrard 2017).

Reviewers may be tempted to save time by only recording the first author followed by "et al."; however, taking the time to record all authors listed can prove to be extremely beneficial.

Although an author may not be the first author on a paper, it is quite possible that they served as the lead author on subsequent publications. By including all authors on the paper, the reviewer is more easily able to track scholars studying and writing about their topic of interest (Garrard 2017). At first glance, date of publication might only seem to be a minor detail. Yet, this simple data point allows the reviewer to understand the historical evolution of a topic. Lastly, it is essential to abstract information about the purpose of the publication. Because IRs include the synthesis of research from diverse methodologies including non-research literature such as theoretical papers, the reviewer needs to understand the researchers' or authors' intent for each source at the start of data abstraction.

Creating the other column topic headings across the top of the review matrix is up to the discretion of the reviewer (Garrard 2017). Some of the more common column topics used are descriptive information about study methods (design, setting, sample, data collection), key results or findings, and quality appraisal data (Booth 2012). The selection of column topics needs to be thoughtfully done. A common mistake novice reviewers make is abstracting data without discernment. The matrix can only help the reviewer with data analysis if the information abstracted from each source is closely aligned with the purpose of the review. It is helpful to include the review purpose or review questions at the top of the matrix or create more than one matrix if multiple questions are used in the review. This provides the reviewer with a visual cue to confirm that the abstracted data have relevance in answering the stated IR purpose and/or questions. A review matrix with an abundance of data unrelated to the review purpose can needlessly complicate the analysis process.

Coughlin and Sethares (2017) provide an excellent example of a review matrix that is closely aligned with the IR purpose and review questions. The purpose of their review was to synthesize the findings of studies on chronic sorrow in parents. The three questions that guided the review were: "(1) How does the experience of chronic sorrow differ between mothers and fathers? (2) What factors have been identified to impact the experience of chronic sorrow overtime? (3) What strategies by healthcare providers for helping parents cope with chronic sorrow have been identified to be most and least helpful?" (p. 109).

Table 5.1 Review matrix with abstracted data aligned with review question: Coughlin and Sethares (2017)

How does the experience of chronic sorrow differ between mothers and fathers?

Author(s)	Year	Method	Sample	Quality rating	Results
Fraley	1986	Mixed method	$N = 36$ parents	Fair	50% of mothers felt depressed; fathers did not; mothers felt higher degree of emptiness, fear of child's future, and guilt. Fathers felt hope
Damrosch and Perry	1989	Close-ended survey	$N = 18$ fathers; $N = 22$ mothers	Good	Nearly all experienced chronic sorrow, not significantly higher for mothers than fathers in total sample, but significant difference for mothers compared with fathers in mother–father pairs Adjustment depicted by fathers as a steady, gradual incline and time-bound, while mothers reported peaks and valleys and/or chronic, periodic crises
Hummel and Eastman	1991	Mixed method	$N = 103$ parents (42 couples; 2 fathers; 17 mothers)	Fair	Many significant differences between mothers and fathers with maternal frequencies almost always greater than paternal on these feelings: crying easily, depression, blaming self, anger, hurt, frustration fear, and others
Hobdell and Deatrick	1996	Mixed method	$N = 132$ (68 mothers and 64 fathers)	Good	Mother's responses were more intense. Mothers: fear and depression; fathers: confusion. Mothers reported more concerns related to social situations. Mothers reported more sorrow and greater intensity. Fathers showed more concerns about future problems and stigma with physical disabilities

Coughlin and Sethares (2017) abstracted data into three separate review matrices. Each review matrix corresponded to the review questions. Table 5.1 illustrates the set up used for the first review question: "How does the experience of chronic sorrow differ between mothers and fathers?" (p. 109). In this table, the review question is explicitly displayed at the top of the table, and the findings column only presents data that specifically relates to how the experience of chronic sorrow differs between mothers and fathers.

Tables 5.2 and 5.3 similarly display the review question at the top of the corresponding review matrix. These tables also demonstrate the use of column headings thoughtfully created to help reviewers' abstract valuable data aligned with the overall purpose and review questions. For example, the main column heading *Factors that led to a resurgence and pervasiveness of chronic sorrow* was further described by using four additional column subheadings and abstracting data related to developmental issues, healthcare related, internal triggers, and lifestyle challenges (Table 5.2). In Table 5.3, Coughlin and Sethares (2017) utilized the main column headings: *strategies most helpful and strategies least helpful*. These column headings were intentionally created to abstract data that is directly aligned with the third review question.

Most novice reviewers are surprised at how tedious and time-consuming abstracting information from each source is (Garrard 2017). Knafl and Whittemore (2017) caution that undertaking a literature review requires patience and perseverance and importantly cannot be rushed. To decrease bias, it is preferable to have more than one reviewer abstract data and to do so independently. The review team would subsequently establish agreement regarding the data abstracted into the review matrix. The benefits of fully engaging in the creation of a review matrix and abstracting process far exceed the time commitment it requires. Our brains can only assimilate information from a few sources of literature at one time (Booth 2012). Through the abstracting process, the reviewer begins to "create order out of chaos" and ownership of the literature (Garrard 2017, p. 140). By taking apart and abstracting information from each source in the sample, the reviewer comes to understand what is known and unknown about the topic of interest, how the phenomenon has evolved, and sets the stage for additional data analysis efforts which compare findings across the body of literature (Whittemore and Knafl 2005; Garrard 2017; Knafl and Whittemore 2017).

5.2.2   Data Analysis Methods

The data analysis stage of the IR requires the reviewer to order, code, and categorize data from multiple sources that may have used diverse methodological perspectives (Whittemore and Knafl 2005; Cooper 1998). A well-done IR meets the same standards as primary research with regard to clarity, rigor, and replication (Beyea and Nicoll 1998). An important question a reviewer should ask when deciding to conduct an IR is: What methods will I use to compare data across studies? (Knafl and Whittemore 2017). An a priori analysis plan and thorough record of all data analysis

Table 5.2 Review matrix with column subheadings: Coughlin and Sethares (2017)

What factors have been identified to impact the experience of chronic sorrow over time?

Author(s)	Year	Method	Sample	Quality rating	Results			
					Factors leading to resurgence and pervasiveness of chronic sorrow			
					Developmental issues	Healthcare related	Internal triggers	Lifestyle challenges
Wikler	1981	Mixed methods	32 parents	Good	Developmental milestones, school entry, onset of puberty, transition to adult/twenty-first birthday/ guardianship	Health crisis management		
Fraley	1986	Mixed methods	39 mothers, 8 fathers	Fair	Falling behind another child developmentally	Stressor events such as surgery, discovery of another medical problem		Need for daycare manifestation of a behavior problem
Hummel and Eastman	1991	Mixed methods	103 parents	Fair	Developmental delay	Illness of child, surgery, repeated illness, follow-up clinic visit		Need for daycare; behavior problems

Table 5.3 Review matrix with abstracted data and column headings aligned with review question: Coughlin and Sethares (2017)

What strategies by healthcare providers for helping parents cope with chronic sorrow have been identified to be most and least helpful?

Author(s)	Year	Method	Sample	Quality rating	Strategies most helpful			Strategies least helpful
					Providing information	Compassionate care	Providing resources	
Fraley	1986	Descriptive closed and open-ended survey	N = 36 parents	Fair	If healthcare professionals offered more explanations about baby's condition, treatments, and procedures	Recognition by healthcare providers of normalcy of feelings parents were having; more support from healthcare team		
Damrosch and Perry	1989	Close-ended survey	N = 18 fathers; N = 22 mothers	Good	Giving parents positive feedback	Assuming cheerful attitude toward parents; encouraging parents not to dwell on the negative; encouraging expression of sadness; encouraging parents to be strong; allowing parents to be weak	Giving parents chance to escape situation	
Cameron, Snowden and Orr	1992	Descriptive, qualitative, retrospective	N = 63 mothers	Good				Barriers to gaining access to healthcare system and delays in getting appointments

Gravelle	1997	Phenomenological	N = 8 parents	Good	Community education about children with disabilities		Respite care crucial; equipment and assistive devices	Needing to form relationships with numerous healthcare providers; frustration with bureaucracy and method of service allocation
Mallow and Bechtel	1999	Open-ended survey	N = 28 (19 mothers, 9 fathers)	Good		Providing holistic, individualized, family-based care; recognizing differences in adaptation between mothers and fathers; being proactively involved;	Appropriate referrals	"Scaring, blaming, and making parents feel guilty"

decisions are essential to increasing rigor in IRs (Whittemore 2005). As such, reviewers should look to use inductive analysis approaches generally associated with qualitative or mixed-method research (Whittemore and Knafl 2005). Some reviewers will use computer software applications, such as NVivo, to assist with coding and analysis. These qualitative analysis software programs can be a useful tool to help organize data; however, manual coding is also a commonly used and effective approach.

Although there is no definitive data analysis method recommended for this stage of the review, constant comparison, content analysis, and thematic analysis are commonly used approaches in IRs (Hopia et al. 2016). The following section provides an overview of these data analysis approaches and an associated exemplar from published IRs. Novice reviewers are encouraged to refer to seminal writings on qualitative data analysis methods for a more in-depth discussion of the theoretical/philosophical underpinnings and analytical approach.

5.2.2.1 Constant Comparison Method

Whittemore and Knafl (2005) provide the most comprehensive discussion of a systematic analytic method reviewers could use during the data analysis stage of an IR. The constant comparison method consists of four phases: data reduction, data display, data comparison, and conclusion drawing and verification (Whittemore and Knafl 2005; Miles and Huberman 1994a).

The first phase, data reduction, refers to the process of selecting, focusing, simplifying, and abstracting data from the sample of primary sources (Whittemore and Knafl 2005; Miles and Huberman 1994a). Data reduction focuses and organizes the data from the primary sources in such a way that the results of the review can be both drawn and verified (Miles and Huberman 1994a). The primary sources in the sample will be initially reduced into subcategories (Whittemore and Knafl 2005). The classification of subcategories is chosen by the reviewer to align with the purpose of the review and facilitate analysis (Whittemore and Knafl 2005). For example, Coughlin and Sethares (2017) created the subcategories providing information, compassionate care, and resources for strategies most helpful for parents coping with chronic sorrow. This data reduction phase reduced a broader category into smaller groupings, which allowed the data to be more focused and detailed.

Data display allows for a compressed presentation of the information from the sample and facilitates conclusion drawing (Miles and Huberman 1994a). Miles and Huberman (1994a) argue that humans are not successfully able to process large amounts of information at one time, and therefore, it is necessary to reduce data into simplified configurations. These configurations can be in the form of grafts, charts, networks, or, as most frequently used, matrices (Miles and Huberman 1994a). It may be necessary to assemble several different matrices to align with the subcategories assembled during data reduction (Whittemore and Knafl 2005). All of these visual displays help the reviewer see what relationships or patterns are emerging within and across the sample of literature (Whittemore and Knafl 2005).

Data reduction and data display are similar to the construction of a review matrix as previously described (Garrard 2017). An important point is that data reduction and data display are not merely steps in preparation of analysis; they are an essential part of the analysis (Miles and Huberman 1994a). These crucial first phases of analysis allow a reviewer to process a large amount of information from the sample and begin to synthesize the body of literature.

The data comparison phase involves examining the data displays for patterns, themes, commonalities, and differences across the review sample (Whittemore and Knafl 2005). This phase can feel overwhelming, but starting with a "squint analysis" by examining where the review matrix looks sparse or dense can begin to highlight patterns across the rows (Miles and Huberman 1994b, p. 190). Whittemore and Knafl (2005) outline several strategies to further enhance the identification of patterns, themes, and relationships including clustering, counting, and making contrasts and comparisons. These rigorous analytic activities support the drawing of conclusions during the final phase of the constant comparison method.

Conclusions are the results of the review. Conclusions are conceptualized at a higher level of abstraction by moving inductively from particulars to the general (Whittemore and Knafl 2005). Verification during this final phase is equally important (Miles and Huberman 1994a). The verification process may include a return to the sample sources to confirm truthfulness of the conclusions or may involve the confirmation of the identified patterns, themes, and relationships by colleagues (Whittemore and Knafl 2005; Miles and Huberman 1994a).

Brady et al. (2019, p. 109) used the constant comparison method during the data analysis stage of their IR of woman-centered care:

> Data analysis was undertaken using the four-phase process as described by Whittemore and Knafl (2005). During the first stage (data reduction), data were divided and organised into groups of differing methodologies (qualitative, quantitative) as well as the themes of woman-centred care in clinical practice, maternity service, and education. The second phase (data display) used the NVivo coding system to highlight and collate data from the studies into organised reference coded nodes (NVivo, 2012). The third stage (data comparison) examined the data displays of the primary sources to identify patterns, themes and relationships (Whittemore and Knafl 2005). The qualitative data offered rich descriptions of the woman-centred care concept and were used to identify components of woman-centred care and relationships between the characteristics, behaviours and outcomes of woman-centred care. The quantitative studies were analysed using a similar process with study content, outcomes and findings of the pre-determined themes allocated to themes and subthemes. To support interpretation and provide clarity, the data were also organised into a visual representation (Whittemore and Knafl 2005).The fourth and final stage (conclusion drawing and verification) assisted in developing interpretations, derived from the previous stages, into conclusions or assumptions about the presentation of the concept of woman-centred care in the empirical literature.

5.2.2.2 Content Analysis

Content analysis is a form of analysis used with either qualitative or quantitative data and is orientated toward summarizing the informational content of data (Elo and Kynga 2008; Sandelowski 2000). Inductive content analysis consists of three phases: preparation, organizing, and reporting (Elo and Kynga 2008). During the

Table 5.4 Content analysis: organizing phase (Elo and Kynga 2008)

Open coding	Written material is read and headings are written in the margins to describe content
Coding sheets	All headings written in the margins during open coding are transferred to a coding sheet and initial categories are created
Grouping	Categories are grouped under higher order headings Similar categories are collapsed and dissimilar categories are broadened to create the higher order headings
Categorization	Through interpretation, generate categories to describe the phenomenon of interest
Abstraction	Using content characteristic words, create generic and subcategories to further describe the phenomenon

preparation phase, the reviewer is immersed in the data and is focused on getting a sense of the whole (Elo and Kynga 2008). Sandelowski (1995) suggests that data preparation is a distinct phase of the analysis process where data are put in a form that facilitates analysis. In traditional qualitative data analysis, this often occurs during the proofing of transcribed audio-recorded interviews (Sandelowski 1995). In IRs, data preparation would consist of reading and abstracting data from the primary sources into a review matrix.

During the organizing phase of inductive content analysis, the reviewer moves through a five-step process. The steps include open coding, coding sheets, grouping, categorization, and abstraction (Elo and Kynga 2008). Table 5.4 outlines these steps. The last phase is the reporting phase where the reviewer reports the results of the analysis using models, conceptual systems, conceptual mapping, or categories (Elo and Kynga 2008). The reviewer presents tables to demonstrate the linkages between the data, categories created, and final results. The presentation phase fosters trustworthiness in the data analysis and results (Elo and Kynga 2008).

Cameron et al. (2011, p. 1375) described the use of content analysis during the data analysis stage of their IR:

> Innovatively in this review, qualitative content analysis was used (Sandelowski 2000). This involved reading and re-reading the papers and preparing a short descriptive summary (Table 2). Codes were also generated to enable the findings to be compared within and between the papers. Each paper was analyzed by two reviewers and the codes agreed through review and negotiation.

5.2.2.3 Thematic Analysis

Thematic analysis is a widely used, flexible method for identifying, analyzing, and reporting patterns within data (Braun and Clarke 2006). Although most commonly used in qualitative data analysis, the approach can also be used to identify and organize the main, recurrent, or most important themes or concepts across multiple sources of literature (Popay et al. 2006). In thematic analysis, the reviewer searches across the review matrix to find repeated patterns. If the review was guided by specific review questions, then the analysis would inform or answer these aims by identifying unifying themes. Braun and Clarke (2006) outline a recursive six-phase process, where you move back and forth as needed, to guide the thematic analysis

Table 5.5 Thematic analysis (Braun and Clarke 2006)

Familiarizing with data	Engage in data immersion including reading and rereading, transcribing data, and taking notes regarding initial ideas for coding
Generating initial codes	Produce initial codes that identify interesting information from the data
Searching for themes	Sort the different codes into potential themes and subthemes Create visual representations to help sort codes into themes (tables, mind-maps, theme piles)
Reviewing themes	Refine themes by collapsing or broadening themes that lack data support or data that are too diverse Ensure alignment of coded data with candidate theme and create candidate thematic map Reread the entire data set to determine if the thematic map represents the data set as a whole and add additional codes or recode as needed
Defining and naming themes	Further define and refine themes and determine what aspect of the data each theme captures Identify the overall story each theme tells, decide whether or not a theme contains any subthemes Think about the final theme names that are concise, and immediately give the reader a sense of what the theme is about
Producing the report	Produce a narrative report that tells the story of your data within and across themes Provide sufficient evidence to support the developed themes and assure the reader regarding the validity of the analysis

approach. The six phases include familiarizing yourself with your data, generating initial codes, searching for themes, reviewing themes, defining and naming themes, and producing the report (Braun and Clarke 2006). Table 5.5 presents the six phases and the associated analytic activities.

Tobiano et al. (2015, p. 1110, 1114) provided a thorough description of the thematic data analysis approach used to synthesize nurse and patient perceptions of patient participation in nursing care.

> Thematic synthesis was used for analysing and synthesising the findings of the included studies, using Thomas and Harden's (2008) work as a guide. First, the researcher became immersed in the data by reading and re-reading the sections labelled "results" or "findings" of each article, maintaining notes of possible patterns and decisions throughout the thematic analysis and synthesis. Second, the findings or results sections were analysed inductively. Line by line coding using words was undertaken, with analysis occurring within and across studies. NVivo 10 software (QSR International) was used to assist with data management. Next, inductive codes were grouped into hierarchies of categories and sub-categories, producing largely descriptive categories. Finally, the categories were searched for the latent themes that went beyond the original content of the studies to provide a meta-synthesis.

Strategies for data analysis with IRs are continuously evolving. Despite data analysis methods being the least established stage of the IR process, it is imperative that reviewers use rigorous methods and keep transparent records of all data analysis procedures (Whittemore and Knafl 2005; Whittemore 2005). Reviewers need to provide explicit details during dissemination about approaches used during the data analysis stage, as this essential phase is often only briefly discussed (Hopia et al. 2016). Efforts to utilize systematic methods and report sufficient methodological details enhance the trustworthiness of IRs and the applicability of findings to practice (Whittemore 2005; Toronto et al. 2018).

5.3   Descriptive Results

The results of the IR are presented in a fully integrated report. However, unlike the report format of a research study, there are no established guidelines to structure the report of a review (Torraco 2005). Many reviewers will begin their result section with a comprehensive description of the sample of literature used for the review. Some of the characteristics discussed include, but are not limited to, methodological design, country of origin, and date range of included literature. Review results can be displayed in a table or diagram to assist the reader in clearly seeing the details of included sources and the linkages to synthesized results (Whittemore and Knafl 2005).

5.4   Synthesis

The reviewer should synthesize the information from diverse sources into a coherent understanding of the topic that supports the stated purpose of the review. This is most commonly presented as a narrative or thematic synthesis (Toronto et al. 2018). Knafl and Whittemore (2017) caution against simply describing the details of each individual source of literature, a process referred to as "laundry listing." Synthesis is a complex process; however, vigilant attention during the data analysis stage of the review supports the synthesis of information across multiple sources.

The organization of the synthesis of results is dependent on methodological decisions made during the earlier stages of the review. For example, when reviewers articulate a purpose and/or review question(s), a narrative or thematic synthesis aligned with these options can be presented. Coughlin and Sethares (2017) organized their narrative synthesis to correspond with the three review questions used to guide the review. In contrast to the presentation of this narrative synthesis, an IR on family presence during cardiopulmonary resuscitation presented a thematic synthesis for each of the stated review questions (Toronto and LaRocco 2019). Presenting the results through the use of a framework or model is yet another approach to synthesizing a body of literature (Harstade et al. 2018).

Synthesis within themes continues to be the most common approach to present the results of IRs (Toronto et al. 2018). These themes are developed during the data analysis stage and used as an organizing structure in the results section.

Alexis and Worsley (2018, p. 158) IR exploring the fears of prostate cancer and screening attitudes of black men of African and Caribbean descent describe the development of four themes during the data analysis stage of their review. These themes were presented in a table with associated characteristics and used to organize the synthesis of their findings. The reviewers provide a clear description of their thematic analysis and how their results were presented in relation to the developed themes:

> After completion, these categories were aggregated into synthesized themes which formed the basis of the findings. These emergent themes were knowledge of prostate cancer, fear, personal factors and access to treatment. Figure 2 details the characteristics of each theme. They will be explored in further detail below.

The data analysis stage and synthesis of findings are quite challenging. However, adherence to systematic approaches during this stage of the IR process is essential to mitigating potential bias or errors in interpretation (Whittemore and Knafl 2005). It is only through the execution of rigorous review methods that synthesis of evidence be truly embraced and integrated into practice.

References

Alexis O, Worsley A (2018) An integrative review exploring black men of African and Caribbean backgrounds, their fears of prostate cancer and their attitudes towards screening. Health Educ Res 33(2):155–166. https://doi.org/10.1093/her/cyy001

Beyea SC, Nicoll LH (1998) Writing an integrative review. AORN J 67(4):877–880

Blondy LC, Blakeslee AM, Scheffer BK, Rubenfeld MG, Cronin BM, Luster-Turner R (2016) Understanding synthesis across disciplines to improve nursing education. West J Nurs Res 38(6):668–685

Booth A (2012) Synthesizing included studies. In: Booth A, Papaioannou D, Sutton A (eds) Systematic approaches to a successful literature review. Sage, London, pp 125–169

Brady S, Lee N, Gibbons K, Bogossian F (2019) Woman-centred care: an integrative review of the empirical literature. Int J Nurs Stud 94:107–119

Braun V, Clarke V (2006) Using thematic analysis in psychology. Qual Res Psychol 3(2):77–101. https://doi.org/10.1191/1478088706qp063oa

Cameron J, Roxburgh M, Taylor J, Lauder W (2011) An integrative literature review of student retention in programmes of nursing and midwifery education: why do students stay? J Clin Nurs. 20:1372–1382. https://doi.org/10.1111/j.1365-2702.2010.03336.x

Cooper H (1998) Synthesizing research: a guide for literature reviews, 3rd edn. Sage, Thousand Oaks, CA

Coughlin MB, Sethares KA (2017) Chronic sorrow in parents of children with a chronic illness or disability: an integrative literature review. J Pediatr Nurs 37:108–116

Elo S, Kynga SH (2008) The qualitative content analysis process. J Adv Nurs 62(1):107–115. https://doi.org/10.1111/j.1365-2648.2007.04569.x

Garrard J (2017) Health sciences literature review made easy: the matrix method. In: Chapter 5, Review matrix folder: how to abstract the research literature, 4th edn. Jones & Bartlett Learning, Burlington, MA, pp 139–160

Harstade CW, Blomberg K, Benzein E, Ostland U (2018) Dignity-conserving care actions in palliative care: an integrative review of Swedish research. Scand J Caring Sci 32(1):8–23. https://doi.org/10.1111/scs.12433

Hopia H, Latvala E, Liimatainen L (2016) Reviewing the methodology of an integrative review. Scand J Caring Sci 30:662–669

Knafl K, Whittemore R (2017) Top 10 tips for undertaking synthesis research. Res Nurs Health 40:189–193

Miles MB, Huberman AM (1994a) Chapter 1, Introduction. In: Qualitative data analysis: an expanded sourcebook, 2nd edn. Sage, Thousand Oaks, CA, pp 1–11

Miles MB, Huberman AM (1994b) Chapter 7, Cross-case displays: exploring and describing. In: Qualitative data analysis: An expanded sourcebook, 2nd edn. Sage, Thousand Oaks, CA, pp 172–205

Popay J, Roberts H, Sowden A, Petticrew M, Arai L, Rodgers M, Britten N (2006) Chapter 3, Guidance on narrative synthesis: an overview. In: Guidance on the conduct of narrative synthesis in systematic reviews: a product from the ESRC methods programme. ESRC, pp 11–24

Sandelowski M (1995) Qualitative analysis: what it is and how to begin. Res Nurs Health 18:371–375. https://doi.org/10.1002/nur.4770180411

Sandelowski M (2000) Focus on research methods: whatever happened to qualitative description? Res Nurs Health 23:334–340

Tobiano G, Marshall A, Bucknall T, Chaboyer W (2015) Patient participation in nursing care on medical wards: an integrative review. Int J Nurs Stud 52:1107–1120. https://doi.org/10.1016/j.ijnurstu.2015.02.010

Toronto CE, LaRocco SA (2019) Family perception of and experience with family presence during cardiopulmonary resuscitation: an integrative review. J Clin Nurs 28(1):32–46

Toronto CE, Quinn B, Remington R (2018) Characteristics of reviews published in nursing literature: a methodological review. ANS Adv Nurs Sci 41(1):30–40. https://doi.org/10.1097/ANS.0000000000000180

Torraco RJ (2005) Writing integrative literature reviews: guidelines and examples. Hum Resour Dev Rev 4(3):356–367

Torraco RJ (2016) Writing integrative literature reviews: using the past and present to explore the future. Hum Resour Dev Rev 15(4):404–428. https://doi.org/10.1177/1534484316671606

Whittemore R (2005) Combining evidence in nursing research: methods and implications. Nurs Res 54(1):56–62

Whittemore R, Knafl K (2005) The integrative review: updated methodology. J Adv Nurs 52(5):546–553. https://doi.org/10.1111/j.1365-2648.2005.03621.x

Discussion and Conclusion

6

Coleen E. Toronto and Ruth Remington

Contents

6.1	Writing the Discussion Section.	72
	6.1.1 Audience.	73
	6.1.2 Fundamental Structure.	73
	6.1.3 Beginning the Discussion Section.	73
6.2	Interpretation of Findings.	75
	6.2.1 Comparison to Background Literature.	75
	6.2.2 Comparison to Theoretical Framework.	76
	6.2.3 Comparison to Similar Research.	77
	6.2.4 Unexpected Findings.	77
6.3	Implications.	77
	6.3.1 Research.	78
	6.3.2 Practice.	78
	6.3.3 Education.	79
	6.3.4 Policy.	79
6.4	Limitations.	79
	6.4.1 Limitations of the Review.	80
	6.4.2 Limitations of Literature Included in Reviews.	80
6.5	Conclusion.	82
6.6	Summary Points.	82
6.7	Conclusion.	83
References.		83

C. E. Toronto (✉)
School of Nursing, Curry College, Milton, MA, USA
e-mail: ctoronto0712@curry.edu

R. Remington
Department of Nursing, Framingham State University, Framingham, MA, USA

© Springer Nature Switzerland AG 2020
C. E. Toronto, R. Remington (eds.), *A Step-by-Step Guide to Conducting an Integrative Review*, https://doi.org/10.1007/978-3-030-37504-1_6

6.1   Writing the Discussion Section

The discussion section is the heart of any scientific paper. This is where new thoughts and directions are introduced and where reviewers provide context and meaning to their research findings (Hess 2004). Some suggest that the discussion is the most difficult part of a literature review to write (Aveyard 2019) and that it demands the most effort and critical thinking of reviewers (Kearney 2017).

The goal of an integrative review (IR) is the development of a holistic understanding of the topic of interest by presenting the state of the science and theoretical and practical consequences of review findings. Skelton and Edwards (2000) propose that reviewers should go beyond the evidence and reach a conclusion that is not found in the results. The discussion is the part of the review where subjective perspectives of reviewers are justified and necessary.

Reviewers' expert knowledge based on previous clinical and research experiences informs the discussion. For these reasons writing the discussion can be challenging. To advance reviewers' understanding of what should be included in this part of an integrative review, this chapter recommends a fundamental structure to follow when writing the discussion section and provides writing examples that demonstrate specific elements of an integrative IR discussion.

The discussion offers an explanation of the findings of the synthesis. New findings should not be presented in the discussion but should be described in the results section. It is unnecessary to develop a discussion section if reviewers simply repeat the main findings of their review without offering interpretation. It is important to emphasize that the discussion presents an interpretation of the review results and the significance and importance to the discipline.

The IR is a distinctive form of research that uses existing literature to create new knowledge (Torraco 2016). The discussion should clearly highlight how the review addressed the gap in the literature that was identified in the introduction section and how the findings and conclusions of the review extend what is known about the phenomenon of interest (Flanagan 2018; Oermann and Hays 2019).

Ghazal and colleagues's (2019, p. 32) review of international educated nurses' experiences in transitioning to nursing practice in the United States provides an example of how reviewers addressed a gap in nursing literature and how their analysis of review findings extends the state of nursing science:

> This study contributes to the growing body of syntheses surrounding international educated nurses (IEN) transition to practice (TTP) experiences and suggests that IENs experience social and cultural transitions that further challenge their vulnerability. This study makes a new contribution to the literature by synthesizing the facilitators and barriers marked in IENs' TTP in the United States, which has been missing, and highlights areas that can be targeted by current and future TTP programs across the United States.

6.1.1 Audience

Hess (2004) advises reviewers to write the discussion for the potential reader, whereas Watson (2018) directs reviewers to write the discussion for editors and peer reviewers. Both of these approaches should be followed. Ultimately, all readers of the review need to find value in the findings of the review in the context of what is known, new knowledge generated, and what is needed in future research. There is no particular modus operandi for reviewers to follow when writing the discussion section (Watson 2018). Likewise, journal publication requirements may differ. To address this uncertainty, it is recommended that reviewers locate examples of published reviews in the targeted journal to which they plan to submit. Generally, these publications provide discussion formats that are preferred by the journal editor and manuscript reviewers of the intended journal (Watson 2018).

6.1.2 Fundamental Structure

Despite variations in published discussion formats, there is a fundamental structure to follow when writing a discussion for an IR. A model often used in scientific writing demonstrates a dynamic relationship between the introduction and discussion sections of a scientific paper. The introduction part of the scientific paper has been illustrated as an inverted triangle and the discussion section is visualized as a triangle. Consequently, the introduction and discussion when combined form an hourglass shape. This is known as the hourglass model within scientific writing circles (Schulte 2003) (Fig. 6.1).

The process of developing the introduction section of a review was addressed in a previous chapter. The hourglass model highlights the symbiotic relationship between the introduction and discussion sections of a review. The introduction section starts broadly with a discussion of the IR topic and narrows to the purpose and/ or review question(s). Conversely, the discussion section starts narrowly with presenting summarized findings that answer the IR's review question(s), and then widens making comparisons with background literature and review findings within the wider context of the literature on the topic. A typical discussion section consists of summary of major findings; comparison of these findings with the introduction's background literature and literature reported elsewhere (conclusions); IR's strengths and limitations; and implications for practice (Cals and Kotz 2013), research, and/ or theory, education, and policy.

6.1.3 Beginning the Discussion Section

The literature reveals differing opinions on how to begin the discussion section (Kearney 2017; Watson 2018). At the outset, Rousch (2019) and Coughlan and

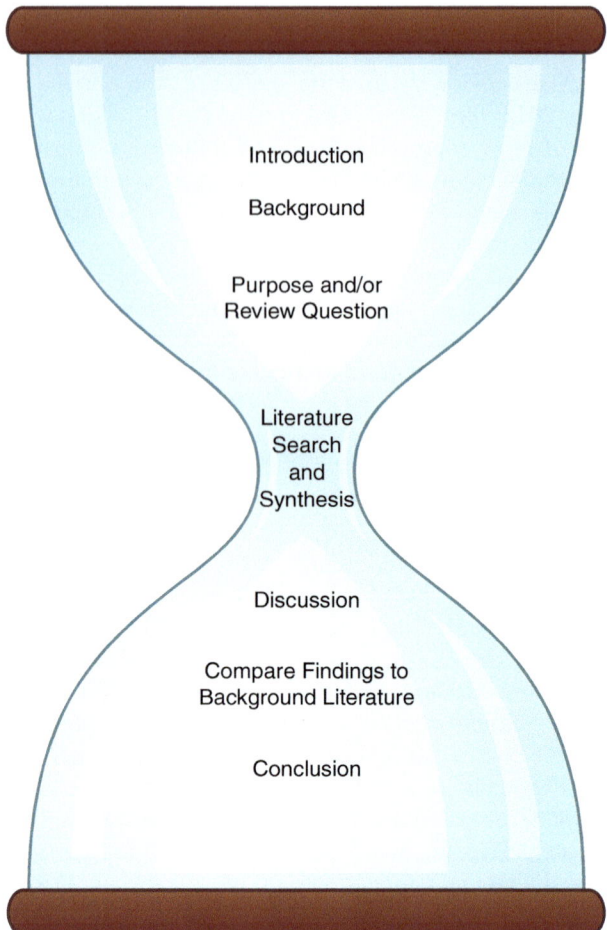

Fig. 6.1 Hourglass model

Cronin (2017) recommend that the beginning of the discussion restates the purpose of the review to remind readers of what question(s) the review answers. This will inform readers about how the discussion section connects back to the introduction of the review. After restating the purpose, the discussion generally provides a brief summary (one to two paragraphs) of major findings (Connelly 2009). The key findings should relate to the purpose/review question(s) of the review.

Stamp and colleagues' (2014, p. 150) IR examined the impact of transitional care programs on adults with heart failure and healthcare organizations and provides a succinct one paragraph summary of major findings after explicitly restating the IR's purpose:

The purpose of this review was to synthesize the literature relating to transitional care programs for heart failure (HF) patients and the effects of these programs on hospital readmission rates, quality of life (QOL), and cost-effectiveness. Comparisons of transitional care programs identified a gap in the literature pertaining to transitional care in HF patients as well as the great variability in the programs that have been studied.

6.2   Interpretation of Findings

After summarizing the major findings, the hourglass model broadens to present the interpretation of review findings. Discussion of findings is made by comparing and contrasting the findings of the review to background literature in the introduction, the theoretical framework of the review (if used), and those of similar research (Bettany-Saltikov 2010). The comparison of similarities and differences between the review findings and the literature provides context and clarity to conclusions that will follow.

The reviewer has the opportunity to provide their interpretations of the meaning and importance of the findings as long as these comments can be compared to existing literature (Coughlan and Cronin 2017). Interpretation is a subjective endeavor. Therefore, reviewers should avoid reading more into review findings than can be supported by the literature. During the development of this part of the discussion section, any statements made by reviewers regarding relationships and how these findings are incorporated into the wider context of the state of science require deliberate reflection and support from primary sources to avoid premature or inaccurate conclusions of accumulated evidence (de Souza et al. 2010).

The discussion may be organized by discussing findings as they relate to the review question(s) or if used guiding theoretical framework. Each review question should have some discussion that provides interpretation of related findings.

6.2.1   Comparison to Background Literature

In this stage of the discussion process, comparisons are made between the synthesized theoretical literature presented in the introduction and the interpretation of findings found in the discussion (de Souza et al. 2010). This relationship between the discussion and introduction sections is highlighted in the hourglass model (Fig. 6.2).

White et al.'s (2019, p. 124) IR identified and assessed evidence regarding self-efficacy for management of symptoms and symptom distress in adults with cancer. In the following paragraph, their discussion connected key review findings back to Bandura's self-efficacy theory presented in the background and significance section of their review:

> This encompassed coaching and education regarding symptom management tailored to the patient's situation, return demonstrations of skills, and ensuring mechanisms for adults to communicate and discuss presence of symptoms. These are all effective strategies for enhancing self-efficacy for symptom management and are consistent with Bandura's (1997) self-efficacy theory.

Fig. 6.2 Relationship
between introduction and
discussion sections

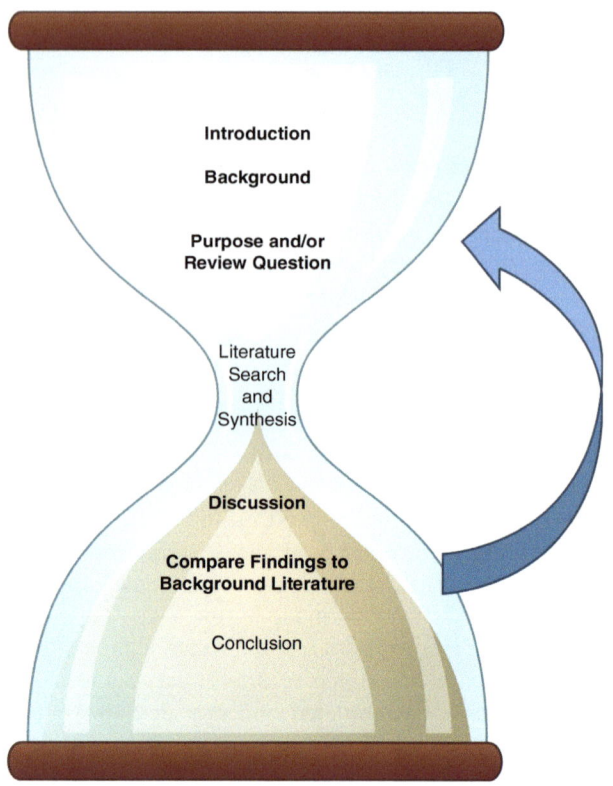

6.2.2   Comparison to Theoretical Framework

If a theoretical framework was used to guide the IR, then reviewers could organize
their discussion around that framework. Rousch (2019) provides three options to
consider when using a theoretical framework to organize a discussion section: (1)
summarize in one to two paragraphs how the findings connect to the theoretical
framework, (2) organize the discussion using the key concepts of the theoretical
framework, and (3) assimilate statements throughout the discussion how particular
findings relate to the theoretical framework and identify any theoretical
implications.

An example of an IR that used a theoretical framework can be found in Gibbons,
Ross, and Bevan's (2014, p. 432) IR in which Van Gennep's (1961) rite of passage
theoretical model and Turner's definition of liminality (1994) were used to organize
their review. Below these reviewers make explicit connections to the theoretical
framework used when summarizing review findings in their discussion section:

> In this integrative review, the transition to family caregiving was characterized as a liminal
> experience occurring in the phases of a rite of passage… Caregivers universally experi-
> enced an event that resulted in the need to respond with a commitment to care for their
> loved one (pre-liminal phase), followed by a period of transition when life as they previously

experienced it, including social roles and relationships, had changed (liminal phase); this period was steeped in uncertainty and suffering. Eventually, caregivers reincorporated the disease or disability into their lives (post-liminal phase), and some even experienced growth and found meaning.

Throughout the remainder of the discussion, Gibbons, Ross, and Bevans (2014) provide statements on how particular review findings relate to the review's guiding theoretical framework.

6.2.3   Comparison to Similar Research

When multiple research studies provide results that lead to similar conclusions, reviewers draw broader understanding of the phenomenon under investigation. Brady et al. (2019, p. 116) conducted an IR to explore, review, and synthesize the empirical literature that reports on the concept of woman-centered care. The reviewers compared and contrasted literature within their review to broader literature, which was not part of the review sample, to demonstrate similarities and differences of the review findings.

> Many of the studies included in this review confirm that the concept of woman-centered care is fundamental to, and a cornerstone of, good midwifery practice… In the broader literature, the aspects of the provision of choice and control for the woman and her family during pregnancy and birth are considered paramount to both physical and psychological well-being. These ideas have long been understood, with earlier studies identifying that women who experienced social aspects of maternity care, for example, the development of relationships, continuity of carer, and having choice and control, had greater satisfaction with their individual experiences…

6.2.4   Unexpected Findings

Reviewers should discuss any unexpected findings found in the review and consider alternative explanations of the findings. When discussing an unexpected finding, begin the paragraph with the finding and then describe it. Lee et al. (2019, p. 296) published an IR that examined the relationships between safety culture and patient safety and quality of care outcomes in hospital settings and provide a discussion example of considering alternative explanations:

> The most notable finding of this review was the large quantity of inconsistencies involving nonsignificant relationships present in the studies … Many factors could have contributed to these inconsistent results, including methodological variations, infrequent use of a theory or theoretical framework, limited discussions of validity of instruments.

6.3   Implications

After reviewers compare review findings against the introduction's background literature and other literature, the hourglass model remains broaden. Reviewers should formulate recommendations or implications for research, practice, education, theory, and/or policy as appropriate. Not all domains will need to be addressed. Implications formulated for research, practice, or other domains will depend on the purpose of the IR and the aims of the journal considered for submission (Bowman 2007).

6.3.1 Research

Although a review may address certain aims or review questions, other review questions may emerge related to the topic. After identifying gaps in knowledge, it is possible to set research priorities for future studies. A major aim of an IR is to make suggestions for further research (de Souza et al. 2010). Rückholdt et al. (2019, p. 50) conducted an IR to examine the complexity of coping and its impact on family members in the ICU environment. Reviewers formulated and proposed research implications in their discussion:

> Further clarification is needed of the specific contribution of coping strategies by family members to their health and well-being. Comparison of family members recruited from non-ICU settings may also help reveal different choices and usage of coping strategies in contrast to the ICU-setting findings presented in this review. This may also help to extend identification of predictors of perceived coping effectiveness by family members. Longitudinal studies are needed to evaluate the effectiveness of coping over time that may help determine the best timing for intervention approaches aimed to help family members adapt and cope with the hospitalisation experience as well as capture the potential dynamism of coping. Additionally, future studies should focus on determining what other modifiable factors could be instigated by the healthcare team in the ICU and post ICU hospital environment to promote adaptive coping responses and promote wellbeing of family members during this stressful period.

6.3.2 Practice

Clearly stated implications for clinical practice, supported by strong evidence, help to support evidence-based nursing and improve the quality of patient care. Cooper and Compton (2019, p. 397) identify the clinical relevance of their review findings by providing practice implications for psychiatric-mental health (PMH) nurses:

> No nursing intervention can happen without nursing assessment. Initiating the conversation on sexual dysfunction (SD) and creating space for patients to voice their concern is still important even when discussing interventions. A question as simple as "any sexual dysfunction?" may suffice or, for a more detailed assessment, the PMH nurse can administer validated tools for SD (such as those mentioned previously in this review). This step in the nursing process may be where PMH nurses are exceptionally skilled. PMH nurses frequently care for patients with histories of trauma, substance abuse, and suicidal behaviors; all of which are difficult topics to discuss. Yet, PMH nurses therapeutically use themselves to create a sense of safety and explore these sensitive issues. Talking about and assessing for SD, even in the absence of any symptoms, can be a powerful intervention where the nurse effectively "leaves the door open". Doing this, the PMH nurse lets the patient know that they are a concerned professional who welcomes a discussion on SD and the totality of sexual health.

6.3.3 Education

Considering the findings of the review and the aims of the targeted journal, educational implications may be warranted. An IR by Foster and colleagues (2018, p. 3) synthesized literature on how simulation is used to teach teamwork skills to pre-licensure nursing students. Educational implications were presented in their discussion:

> Because situation awareness and leadership skills studies were lacking in this review, nurse educators should revise their simulation curriculum to effectively teach these skills to students. One suggestion is the use of valid and reliable tools such as the Situation Awareness Global Assessment Technique and Team-Assessment Inventory to help educators determine if students are gaining knowledge about these concepts. The authors also suggest using the TeamSTEPPS framework when developing simulation objectives to ensure inclusion of key concepts. In addition, educators should ensure that they are adhering to standards of simulation, which includes debriefing using constructivist methods. This type of debriefing could be helpful for enhancing teamwork skills.

6.3.4 Policy

Policy implications while not often found in nurse-authored IRs can be an important implication to consider for some review topics. Toronto and LaRocco's (2019, p. 13) IR focused on family perceptions and experiences of family presence during resuscitation (FPDR). Reviewers provided policy implications for nurses to consider when addressing family presence during resuscitation (FPDR) in the hospital setting:

> Our healthcare culture has moved to more patient-centered care, with an emphasis on family involvement. However, healthcare systems do not automatically default to allowing FPDR …Instead, patients' family members are all too often ushered into a waiting room to await being updated about the outcome of the resuscitation efforts of their family member… To address this issue, clear policies that support the option, not mandate, of FPDR as a patient-centered practice, and trained HCPs are needed for the implementation of FPDR. This would help to alleviate the disparities that are caused by different staff members' opinion as to what is right in a code situation. This hospital-based policy initiative is supported by professional organisations such as the Emergency Nurses Association for more than 20 years. (Emergency Nurses Association 2010)

6.4 Limitations

Reviewers should discuss the limitations of their IR in the discussion section. This is not a review of the limitations of individual studies (which was completed during the critical appraisal process), but a review of the limitations of the review itself. When reviewers are explicit in identifying the limitations of the review, it is often viewed as more credible and ultimately strengthens the impact of the review (Coughlan and Cronin 2017). The results of an IR may be limited by the flaws of the selected studies, by the weaknesses of the review itself or both. As with any research study, all reviews have methodological shortcomings that cannot be overcome; however, there is a need to acknowledge these to readers. It is best if limitations are identified by reviewers of the review rather than peer reviewers or editors that point out the review's methodological issues.

In addition to weaknesses, strengths of the review should be noted (Coughlan and Cronin 2017). Reviewers are encouraged to critically ponder the overall review strengths and weaknesses of their review and of the included literature (Robertson-Malt 2014). Critical reflection by reviewers looking back on the process of conducting the review will assist in identifying limitations. The noted limitations should have a subheading to alert readers where it is located in the discussion.

6.4.1 Limitations of the Review

It has been found in nursing literature that published IRs demonstrate a wide variation of how reviewers report their limitations. Hopia and colleagues (2016) examined the methodology used in 10 IRs published in high-impact factor nursing journals. Findings revealed that some reviewers focused only on certain methodological areas of their reviews such as inclusion/exclusion criteria used or quality of data, while others concentrated on wider range of limitations such as cultural factors, quality assessment of study design of individual studies, language restrictions of publications, and how many reviewers participated in a review.

Potential review limitations encountered by reviewers while conducting an IR may relate to potential biases as a result of including only published works, utilizing non-exhaustive search methods due to resource restrictions, or having only a single reviewer. Other limitations may be from the employed search strategy used or the inability to generalize review findings.

Tables 6.1 and 6.2 give examples of weaknesses and strengths of IRs noted in the discussion sections of several reviews published in nursing.

6.4.2 Limitations of Literature Included in Reviews

Critical appraisal of included studies should be included in the results section; however, a summary of the methodological weaknesses of included studies can also be noted in the discussion. White et al. (2019, p. 125) noted these in their limitation section of their IR which examined current literature that addressed self-efficacy for the management of symptoms and symptom distress or frequency and severity in adults with cancer:

> The cross-sectional methodology of some of the articles is also a limitation because self-efficacy has the potential to change depending on phase of treatment and severity of symptoms. Power analysis was frequently omitted from the studies and included in only six of the publications. Although the randomized controlled trials were not blinded to assignment, blinding would be difficult with this type of intervention research.

Table 6.1 Examples of review limitations

Methodological	Reviewer(s)	Example
Search		
Search terms	Coughlin, Sethares (2017, p. 115)	"A potential limitation of this review relates to the search strategy. The search terms of chronic sorrow and parents could have led to missing studies that discussed the same phenomenon but that used other related terms such as grief, depression or sadness"
Search criteria	Lee et al. (2019, p. 300)	"…this review included only studies published in English, and this approach may have excluded relevant evidence published in other languages"
Generalizability	Ghazal et al. (2019, p. 33)	"…there is a lack of studies of international educated nurses (IENs) from certain regions, such as the Middle East, thus our findings may not be generalized to this IEN population"
Single screener and appraiser	Radbron et al. (2019, p. 75)	"The limitations of this review include having a single reviewer screen and appraise the quality of the articles selected…"
Quality appraisal process	Coughlan and Sethares (2017, p. 115)	"Methodologic limitations include using an appraisal tool developed decades after some of the reviewed studies were published. This may have led to erroneously lower appraisal scores on some reports given the standards for writing research reports has evolved over that time period"

Table 6.2 Examples of review strengths

Methodological	Reviewer(s)	Example
Theoretical framework	Gibbons et al. (2014, p. 434)	"The theoretical orientation of the review informed the decisions made in identifying and combining qualitative studies to achieve the goals of this review"
Search criteria	Cartwright et al. (2017, p. 353)	"Establishment of specific inclusion and exclusion criteria and mapping of article selection minimized bias"
Sources	Toronto and LaRocco (2019, p. 14)	"…the use of comprehensive databases and ancestry searches provided a thorough review of the research that has been done related to family perception of and experience with family presence during resuscitation"
Quality appraisal tools	Teunissen et al. (2019, p. 21)	"Validated appraisal tools were applied and all three reviewers appraised the data individually to prevent bias"
Librarian involvement	Classen et al. (2019, p. 9)	"The search strategy was implemented by the health science center librarian…"

6.5   Conclusion

The conclusion will be found at the ending of the discussion or as a stand-alone section that follows the discussion section (Oermann and Hays 2019). The conclusion summarizes the main findings without self-plagiarizing or inserting any new findings or ideas. Consequently, there should be no inclusion of citations (Watson 2018; Dawidowicz 2010). Hess (2004) points out that it is important to highlight key points that the reader will remember from reading the review. Hooker and colleagues' (2015, p. 561) IR synthesized literature on the associations between heart failure (HF) patient–caregiver relationship quality and communication and patient and caregiver health outcomes. The authors provide an example of a written conclusion that summarizes the review's main findings with a clear "take-home" message:

> Relationship quality and communication are associated with the health and well-being of HF patients and their informal family caregivers. However, it is unclear how these factors are related to improved health and wellbeing in both patients and caregivers. Future research should continue to include perspectives of diverse samples of both patients and caregivers to better explain the mechanisms accounting for the associations between relationship quality and communication and heart failure (HF) patient and caregiver health and well-being. In addition, efficacy trials testing interventions to improve patient caregiver relationship quality and communication would provide causal evidence that relationship quality and communication improve patient-caregiver health and well-being.

6.6   Summary Points

In summary, the reviewer should be mindful of essential elements to address in a discussion section of an integrative review:

- Provide a brief summary of the review's purpose and major findings.
- State how the review findings contribute to the understanding of a phenomenon or questions(s).
- Interpret the findings in relation to the literature cited in the background section.
- Describe how the findings fit into the present body of nursing knowledge.
- Place the review in the ongoing conversation and context of the current literature by comparing and contrasting the review findings to the work of other authors.
- State how the findings support, enhance, or contrast with prior evidence.
- Identify implications for research, practice, education, and/or policy.

Equally important to note when writing a discussion is to avoid common pitfalls:

- Simply repeating the information in the results section without any interpretation
- Drawing conclusions or formulating implications that cannot be supported by the literature

- Not making connections to the theoretical framework if used to organize the review
- Not discussing the methodological limitations of the review or review's sample
- Not providing implications for nursing practice, research/theory, education, and/ or policy
- Inserting new information/citations in the conclusion section of the review

6.7   Conclusion

The discussion section can answer the "so what" question or why do these results matter. It is where the new knowledge is identified and interpreted for the reader and for the profession. It may be the most difficult to write, but it is the most important, in that it ties together all of the preceding sections and explains the importance and relevance of the results of the review. Relating the findings of the review to supporting literature places the specific details of the results in the broader context of existing literature and can form the basis for generalization of the review findings.

References

Aveyard H (2019) Doing a literature review in health and social care: practical guide, 4th edn. Open University Press, Bethesda, MD, p 153

Bettany-Saltikov J (2010) Learning how to undertake a systematic review: part 2. Nurs Stand 24:47–56

Bowman KG (2007) A research synthesis overview. Nurs Sci Q 20:171–176. https://doi.org/10.1177/0894318407299575

Brady S, Lee N, Gibbons K, Bogossian F (2019) Woman-centered care: an integrative review of empirical literature. Int J Nurs Stud 94:107–119. https://doi.org/10.1016/j.ijnurstu.2019.01.001

Cals JWL, Kotz D (2013) Effective writing and publishing scientific papers, part VI: Discussion. J Clin Epidemiol 66:1064. https://doi.org/10.1016/j.jclinepi.2013.04.017

Cartwright J, Atz T, Newman S, Mueller M, Demirci JR (2017) Integrative review of interventions to promote breastfeeding in the late preterm infant. JOGN Nurs 46:347–355. https://doi.org/10.1016/j.jogn.2017.01.006

Classen S, Winter SM, Brown C, Morgan-Daniel J, Medhizadah S, Agarwal N (2019) An Integrative Review on teen distracted driving for model program development. Front Public Health [Internet]. Frontiers Media SA 3:7. https://doi.org/10.3389/fpubh.2019.00111

Connelly LM (2009) The discussion section of a research report. Medsurg Nurs 18:300–301

Cooper SA, Compton PA (2019) Nursing interventions for sexual dysfunction: an integrative review for the psychiatric nurse. Arch Psychiatr Nurs 33:389–399. https://doi.org/10.1016/j.apnu.2019.04.003

Coughlan M, Cronin P (2017) Doing a literature review in nursing, health and social care. Sage, London, UK, p 120

Coughlin MB, Sethares KA (2017) Chronic sorrow in parents of children with a chronic illness or disability: an integrative literature review. J Pediatr Nurs 37:108–116. https://doi.org/10.1016/j.pedn.2017.06.011

Dawidowicz P (2010) Literature reviews made easy: a quick guide to success. Information Age Publishing, Charlotte, NC, p 150 de Souza MT, da Silva MD, de Carvalho R (2010) Integrative review: what is it? How to do it? Einstein (São Paulo) 8:102–106. https://doi.org/10.1590/s1679-45082010rw1134

Flanagan J (2018) The integrative review. Int J Nurs Knowl. Wiley 29(2):81. https://doi.org/10.1111/2047-3095.12208

Foster M, Gilbert M, Hanson D, Whitcomb K, Graham C (2018) Use of simulation to develop teamwork skills in prelicensure nursing students: an integrative review. Nurse Educ 44:E7–E11. https://doi.org/10.1097/NNE.0000000000000616.

Ghazal LV, Ma C, Squires A (2019) Transition-to-U.S. practice experiences of internationally educated nurses: an integrative review. West J Nurs Res 4:193945919860855. https://doi.org/10.1177/0193945919860855

Gibbons SW, Ross A, Bevans M (2014) Liminality as a conceptual frame for understanding the family caregiving rite of passage: an integrative review. Res Nurs Health 37:423–436. https://doi.org/10.1002/nur.21622

Hess DR (2004) How to write an effective discussion. Respir Care 49:1238–1241

Hooker SA, Grigsby ME, Riegel B, Bekelman DB (2015) The impact of relationship quality on health-related outcomes in heart failure patients and informal family caregivers: an integrative review. J Cardiovasc Nurs 30:552–563. https://doi.org/10.1097/JCN.0000000000000270

Hopia H, Latvala E, Liimatainen L (2016) Reviewing the methodology of an integrative review. Scand J Caring Sci 30:662–669. https://doi.org/10.1111/scs.12327

Kearney MH (2017) The discussion section tells us where we are. Res Nurs Health 40:289–291. https://doi.org/10.1002/nur.21803

Lee SE, Scott LD, Dahinten VS, Vincent C, Dunn Lopez K, Park CG (2019) Safety culture, patient safety, and quality of care outcomes: a literature review. West J Nurs Res 4(2):279–304. https://doi.org/10.1177/019394591774716

Oermann MH, Hays JC (2019) Writing for publication in nursing, 4th edn. Springer, New York, NY, p 118

Radbron E, Wilson V, McCance T, Middleton R (2019) The use of data collected from mhealth apps to inform evidence-based quality improvement: an integrative review. Worldviews Evid Based Nurs 16:70–77

Robertson-Malt S (2014) Presenting and interpreting findings. Am J Nurs 114:49–54

Roush K (2019) A nurse's step-by-step guide to writing a dissertation or scholarly project (2nd ed.). Sigma Theta Tau International (publisher). p 100

Rückholdt M, Toflera GH, Randall S, Buckley T (2019) Coping by family members of critically ill hospitalised patients: an integrative review. Int J Nurs Stud 97:40–54. https://doi.org/10.1016/j.ijnurstu.2019.04.016

Schulte B (2003) Scientific writing & the scientific method: parallel "Hourglass" structure in form & content. Am Biol Teach 65:591–594. https://doi.org/10.2307/4451568

Skelton JR, Edwards SJL (2000) The function of the discussion section in academic medical writing. Br Med J 320:1269–1270

Stamp KD, Machado MA, Allen NA (2014) Transitional care programs improve outcomes for heart failure patients. J Cardiovasc Nurs [Internet]. Ovid Technologies (Wolters Kluwer Health) 29(2):140–154. https://doi.org/10.1097/jcn.0b013e31827db560

Teunissen C, Burrell B, Maskill V (2019) Effective surgical teams: an integrative literature review. West J Nurs Res 41:1–35. https://doi.org/10.1177/0193945919834896

Toronto CE, LaRocco SA (2019) Family perception of and experience with family presence during cardiopulmonary resuscitation: an integrative review. J Clin Nurs 28:32–46. https://doi.org/10.1111/jocn.14649

Torraco RJ (2016) Writing integrative literature reviews: using the past and present to explore the future. Hum Resour Dev Rev 15:404–428. https://doi.org/10.1177/1534484316671606

Watson R (2018) The discussion section of a manuscript. Nurse, vol 28. Author, p 3

White LL, Cohen MZ, Berger AM, Kupzyk AZ, Bierman PJ (2019) Self-Efficacy for management of symptoms and symptom distress in adults with cancer: an integrative review. Oncol Nurs Forum 46:113–128

Dissemination of the Integrative Review

7

Kristen A. Sethares

Contents

7.1 The Integrative Review to Inform Practice, Program Planning, and Policy............... 85
7.2 Writing Up the Integrative Review... 86
    7.2.1 Manuscript Features... 86
7.3 Conference Presentation.. 91
    7.3.1 Submitting an Abstract.. 91
    7.3.2 Podium Presentation.. 91
    7.3.3 Poster Presentation... 94
7.4 Submitting the Integrative Review for Publication....................................... 96
    7.4.1 Selecting a Journal.. 96
    7.4.2 Preparing the Manuscript for Submission..................................... 100
    7.4.3 Manuscript Submission and Review.. 101
7.5 New Approaches for Dissemination of Reviews.. 103
    7.5.1 News Media... 103
    7.5.2 Social Media.. 104
7.6 Future Needs to Update the Integrative Review.. 104
References... 105

7.1 The Integrative Review to Inform Practice, Program Planning, and Policy

Dissemination is the final phase of research. Dissemination of the integrative review (IR) is the planned process of presenting findings to a targeted audience (Merriam Webster Dictionary n.d.). The process of dissemination occurs in a number of forms and depends on the intended audience of the review. Typical dissemination

K. A. Sethares (✉)
College of Nursing and Health Sciences, University of Massachusetts Dartmouth,
North Dartmouth, MA, USA
e-mail: ksethares@umassd.edu

© Springer Nature Switzerland AG 2020
C. E. Toronto, R. Remington (eds.), *A Step-by-Step Guide to Conducting an Integrative Review*, https://doi.org/10.1007/978-3-030-37504-1_7

approaches include peer-reviewed publications, podium, or poster presentations at conferences, professional seminars, social media, and news media. In this chapter, dissemination of the IR is the focus. Integrative reviews are a method of research centered on finding, reviewing, critiquing, and synthesizing research, theoretical, and methodological literature, to develop new perspectives on a topic (Torraco 2016; Whittemore and Knafl 2005). Integrative reviews can be conducted on a topic with a large amount of research or in an emerging area. Reviewed literature can also be organized conceptually or methodologically (Cooper et al. 2009). The goal of an IR is to critically analyze and synthesize diverse literature to advance knowledge in a topical area and can be used to inform practice and program planning. Knowledge gaps identified in the review inform future research especially when discrepancies are discovered. Finally, the audience of an IR can range from scholars to practitioners to policymakers to the general public, thus increasing the scope of usefulness of the IR methodology (Torraco 2016).

7.2 Writing Up the Integrative Review

Methods of completing all types of reviews have evolved and have become a popular form of publication over the past 20 years (Aveyard and Bradbury-Jones 2019). As a result, confusion about describing and reporting the selected method of review has occurred. Moreover, Aveyard and Bradbury-Jones (2019) found lack of clarity in names for reviews, methods, and appraisal processes used in published nursing reviews.

Reviewers critically synthesize what is known about a topic and give direction for future research, practice, and policy. In dissemination of review findings, it is essential to clearly describe search techniques, analysis, appraisal, and synthesis methods to enhance methodological quality.

7.2.1 Manuscript Features

7.2.1.1 Abstract

Abstracts are short summaries of journal articles found at the beginning of the article or a brief summary of a conference presentation. The abstract in a review manuscript should include a brief overview of the introduction/background, purpose, methods, results, and discussion/implications of the review. Guidelines for the headings and number of words or characters to be included in the abstract are found in the *Information for Authors* section of the selected journal or in the submission guidelines for a particular organization where the presentation is being submitted. Abstracts may be structured, with specific headings, or unstructured, written in a continuous narrative format (Oermann and Hayes 2016). An example of a structured abstract is found in an IR by Toronto and LaRocco (2019) and is included in Fig. 7.1.

Objective: The objective was to consider family presence during resuscitation (FPDR) from the perspective of the family member.

Background: FPDR has been a topic of interest internationally since the first report of this practice more than 25 years ago. Worldwide, many studies have provided insight into the perspective of healthcare professionals (HCPs); however, there is limited research on the perspective and experiences of family members.

Design: An integrative review was conducted. An electronic database search was conducted for the years from 1994–2017.

Methods: The Cumulative Index of Nursing and Allied Health Literature (CINAHL), PyschINFO, Academic Search, SocINDEX, PubMed, ProQuest databases and Google Scholar were searched. Search terms were family perceptions, family presence and resuscitation.

Results: Twelve reviews met inclusion criteria. Findings suggest that family members view family presence as a fundamental right. Family members involved in a FPDR experience reported that their presence benefitted the patient and healthcare team. In an international sample of studies, family presence overall was viewed positively by family members and they voiced wanting to be given an option to be pre- sent during a loved one's resuscitation.

Conclusions: Findings support that family members' desire for FPDR; however, the literature reflects that HCPs do not always embrace the practice of FPDR. Stronger educational preparation of nurses and other HCPs related to FPDR is warranted. Policy initiatives include the formulation of policies that allow family presence during resuscitation of a family member.

Relevance to clinical practice: The findings are relevant for a clinical practice that promotes a more family–centered approach to allowing FPDR. Creating policy and providing FPDR education for HCPs based on evidence provide more consistency in clinical practice and help to eliminate the moral distress experienced by clinical nurses forced to make difficult

Fig. 7.1 Example of a structured abstract

The abstract is generally written after the review is complete; however, enough time should be allotted for this important task. The abstract may be the only part of a manuscript reviewed when an initial database search is done to determine if an article is relevant to a reader for clinical or research purposes (Alspach 2017). Abstracts that include jargon, acronyms, or are unfocused can confuse a reader. Abstracts are also the only part of a manuscript sent to potential peer reviewers; therefore, a poorly written abstract may cause a peer reviewer to refuse to complete the review or form a negative opinion of the manuscript, potentially leading to manuscript rejection (Freysteinson and Stankus 2019; Fowler 2015). Finally, poorly written abstracts may cause database indexing errors making the review difficult to find in a database search by other researchers (Alspach 2017).

Abstracts have little space for describing the reasons, processes, and outcomes of an IR with limits typically between 200 and 500 words. As a result, a balance of information between the required sections is necessary. The background section should include two to three concise sentences that highlight what is known about the topic and the reason for the review. The introduction/background should be compelling and concise, with limited jargon, and capture the reader's attention (Sturgeon and Ditadi 2018). Do not assume that abstract reviewers are familiar with the topic, so clear writing is important. The methods section of a review abstract is generally about three to five sentences that explicitly outline the search strategy, appraisal processes, quality ratings, and comparison of selected literature. The results section should briefly summarize the analysis and synthesis of the review in two to three sentences. Finally, the discussion section should link the findings of the review with what is already known and extend the findings with recommendations for practice change, future research, and/or policy. This section will also include two to three sentences. Because of space limitations, review tables/matrices and flow diagrams cannot be included in the abstract.

7.2.1.2 Introduction or Background

In order to grab the reader's attention, it is important to craft an engaging opening sentence by concretely defining what is known about a topic of interest in terms that are understandable to a wide audience (Freysteinson and Stankus 2019). The background/introduction section of the review succinctly summarizes what is known and why the review is needed (Oermann and Hayes 2016). The aim or purpose of the review should be clearly stated at the end of this section in a single declarative sentence. The purpose should flow from ideas presented in the background/introduction. For example, "The aim of this review is to describe the current evidence of factors related to the decision to delay seeking care in heart failure patients and to link delay to outcomes" (Sethares et al. 2015, p. 95).

7.2.1.3 Method

This section includes the detailed steps that were used to complete the IR. It should be written in a manner that demonstrates the rigor of the review.

Define and Name Review Type

The first step is to clearly name the review type as an IR. Then, provide a definition of the IR with a citation to support the definition. Whittemore and Knafl (2005) published a seminal paper in nursing that defined the types of content typically included in an IR as qualitative, quantitative, and theoretical (p. 547). An integration of these designs provides for a more comprehensive analysis and synthesis of topics of interest to nurses, such as concepts, theories, evidence, and methodological issues (p. 548). However, without a clear methodology outlining how the evidence was found, appraised, and analyzed, the review is incomplete. Several authors support the need for a clear description of these components in the review prior to submission of the manuscript (Bougioukas et al. 2019; Moher et al. 2009).

Formulate the Purpose and/or Review Questions

Prior to beginning a review, a clear definition of the problem is necessary. Generally, the problem will include the broad concept(s) or method of interest and the gap the review is intended to fill. In some cases, the review may be related to a theory or research method. In order to perform a search, a question(s) is necessary to guide the search. The review question(s) in an IR tells the reader of the purpose of the review and outlines the specific goals of the review. In many cases, the review question(s) guides the process of the review by determining the key variables of interest that inform inclusion and exclusion criteria. For example, Coughlin and Sethares' (2017) review included a question about gender differences in the experience of chronic sorrow in parents of children with chronic illness or disability (p. 109). This review question led to the formulation of inclusion criteria that specified a population that included parents of children with chronic illness or disability.

Search and Select Literature Systematically

The next step of disseminating the review is describing the process used for searching for appropriate literature to answer conceptual, theoretical, empirical, or methodological question(s). In this section of the review, clearly report any databases that are searched along with the keywords and any limiters. Limiters are parts of the database that limit the scope of the search and include dates, types of articles, populations, and language. A rationale for selected limiters may be necessary. Some journals may have space limitations and prefer a brief table that summarizes this content rather than writing it up in the manuscript.

Assess the Quality of Selected Literature

Many critical appraisal tools exist to rate the quality of literature included in an IR. A clear description of how the evidence was rated informs the reader about the rigor and quality of the literature included in the review (Bougioukas et al. 2019). Describe the rating tool or tools used to evaluate the quality of the articles included in the review, and include a reference for the tool(s). If a specific tool was not used, clearly articulate the process used to evaluate the quality of the evidence for the reader. Outline the steps used and who was included in the rating process. Numerical or qualitative ratings of the evidence are often included in a column in the summary tables or matrices and used to compare the quality of conflicting findings. These ratings may be useful for making a case for better quality literature in future research and assist readers with determining the best available evidence.

Analyze and Synthesize Literature

Review tables or matrices are used to analyze and synthesize the findings of the review. Tables are generally organized with headings that support analysis and synthesis of literature according to the purpose of the review. Analysis and synthesis have three main goals: "review, update and critique literature, reconceptualize a topic, and answer specific review questions" (Torraco 2016, pp. 411–412).

7.2.1.4 Results

In the search flow diagram, the reviewer will report literature included and excluded from the review. The flow diagram displays the decisions made by the reviewer about which literature was included in the review and the rationale for eliminating an article (Oermann and Hayes 2016). The inclusion and exclusion criteria described

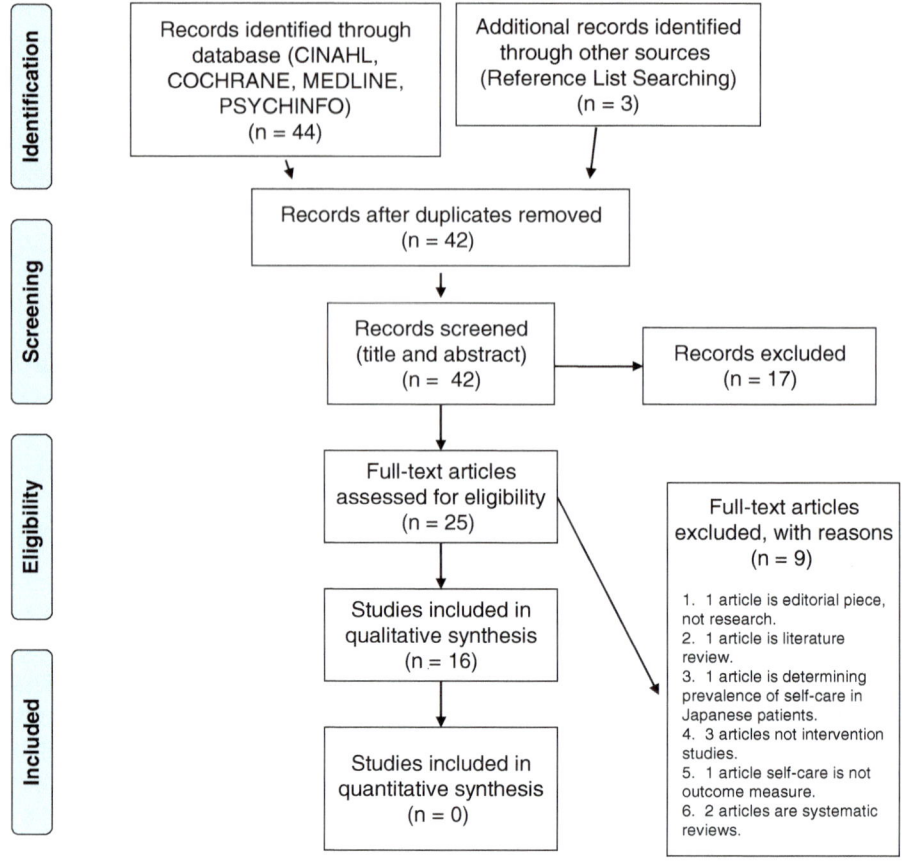

Fig. 7.2 Example of a PRISMA flow diagram

earlier generally guide the choice of what to include and exclude from a review. The number of articles excluded at each step in the process is also listed. Figure 7.2 contains an example of a Preferred Reporting Items for Systematic Reviews and Meta-Analyses (PRISMA) flow diagram that is used to display these decisions (Moher et al. 2009). Finally, analysis and synthesis of the data to answer the review purpose or review question(s) are completed in this section. Useful reviews include a summary of major themes across the reviewed literature rather than a detailed summary of each article reviewed (Oermann et al. 2018).

Houde and Melillo (2002) completed an IR that explored factors influencing physical activity in older adults. This is an excerpt from that study summarizing the findings related to physical activity and blood pressure as an example; "Of the studies that investigated the relationship of physical activity to blood pressure (BP), six studies showed a positive relationship to BP, and three studies showed no relationship to BP. Each of the six studies that evaluated the relationship between physical activity and pulse rate found a decrease in heart rate with increasing physical activity" (p. 227).

7.2.1.5 Discussion

In this section, the main findings are reviewed and linked to what is already known. A critical review of bias and its potential impact on the results are also necessary (Oermann and Hays 2016). Limitations of the review and implications of the findings for practice are included in this section. Recommendations for future research are based on review findings integrated with what is known.

7.2.1.6 References

References are included in the review manuscript according to the guidelines in the *Information for Authors* section of the chosen journal. References for all articles cited in the manuscript should be included in the reference list. References should be current; original; and accurate, and support the points made in the review. The reference list should only include content that was cited in the review. Citation management software may be helpful in formatting reference lists.

7.3 Conference Presentation

7.3.1 Submitting an Abstract

As noted earlier in this chapter, abstracts are brief summaries of completed scholarly work and generally include background/introduction, methods, results, and discussion sections. Guidelines for required headings to include in the abstract are found on the website of the organization where the abstract will be submitted. The conference objectives and the focus of the organization should be reviewed before submitting an abstract to be sure the topic of the review is appropriate for the intended audience. If possible, refer to the conference objectives with one or two keywords in the abstract that link to the focus of the conference. Refer to the earlier section describing what to include in an abstract. An example of a published IR abstract is seen in Fig. 7.3 (Viveiros et al. 2019).

7.3.2 Podium Presentation

Podium presentations are formatted similar to a manuscript. The headings described in the manuscript features section can also be used to guide the development of slides for podium presentation of an IR. Each heading found in the manuscript will be covered on a unique slide and is italicized in this section for ease. The initial side is the *title* and includes the title of the presentation, names of all authors, their credentials, and their respective institutions. *Learning objectives or outcomes* may be a requirement of the organization and should be included after the title slide, if requested. The next slide is the *background/introduction* slide and includes a list of bullet points that summarizes what is the knowledge gap and makes a compelling case for the review. Points on the slide should be referenced using the citation format commonly used in the presenter's discipline. A *reference slide* can be included

Mindfulness-based Interventions in the Heart Failure Population: An Integrative Review

Background: Mild cognitive impairment (MCI), limitations of attention, memory and decision making, creates barriers to treatment adherence and perpetuate inadequate self-care in greater than 50% of heart failure patients. Interventional work focused on improving symptom burden may improve quality of life and reduce morbidity and hospitalization. Mindfulness meditation has recently been viewed as an intervention that may impact cognitive performance and improve HF symptom burden.

Purpose: This integrative review aims to identify and examine current literature on the outcomes of mindfulness-based interventions in the HF population and proposes areas for future study.

Method: The review utilized methods described by Whittemore and Knafl. Three electronic databases (CINAHL, Medline, PsychINFO) were searched from inception through March 2018. The search used the terms "mindfulness OR meditation" and "heart failure" in combination and generated 58 articles after duplicates were removed. Inclusion criteria were: adult HF population; published in English; identified as an empirical study; and mindfulness or meditation as the intervention. Exclusion criteria were: descriptive studies; abstracts; dissertations/editorials; and multi-component interventions, as the specific aspect that contributed to any change could not be determined, eliminating designs using yoga or Tai Chi.

Results: Six studies qualified for review, including four articles with samples from the United States and two articles with samples from Brazil and Sweden, respectively. The total HF patient sample across studies included 320 participants. Interventional design and length varied among the studies, and 20 different dependent variables were identified, ranging from self-reported symptoms to biomarkers. The variation in outcome data limited comparisons across studies.

Conclusion: Mindfulness meditation may provide psychosocial and symptom burden benefits, but data on its impact on cognitive performance is sparse. Opportunities to improve future research should consider: rigorous definition of mindfulness meditation; standardization of intervention characteristics and interventionalist qualifications; more large-scale randomized controlled trials to test theory-driven interventions and linked outcomes; and development of systematic outcome instruments to advance quality evidence for mindfulness interventions in the HF population (19, E 135).

Fig. 7.3 Example of a published abstract of an integrative review

at the end of the presentation. A common mistake made by beginning presenters is including too much information on a slide. Simple bullet points are easier for the audience to read, and the presenter can summarize the details rather than read each bullet point. An example of a background and purpose slide is included in Fig. 7.4. The *purpose* of the review or review question(s) can be listed on the third slide. However, sometimes the purpose is listed at the end of the background section as seen in Fig. 7.4.

For an IR presentation, the methods section of the presentation is divided into several slides rather than a single slide. The *first method* slide will describe the method of the review and would be titled integrative review. On this slide, include a brief description of the chosen method and the process used for finding the literature with keywords, databases, and inclusion and exclusion criteria. On the next *method slide*, presenters should include the process used for critically appraising the

Background and Purpose

- Older heart failure (HF) patients have difficulty recognizing and correctly interpreting symptoms, which can lead to delay in seeking treatment.
- Although symptoms rarely occur in isolation in this population, most predictive models only examine single symptoms in relationship to delay.
- Research has identified symptom clusters in HF, but how these clusters are related to dealy in seeking treatment has not been explicated.
- The purpose of this study is to determine if there are specific symptom clusters predictive of delay in order adults with HF and to further determine if age and gender differences exist in these cluster profiles.

Fig. 7.4 Example of a background and purpose slide for a podium presentation

literature and describe any resources used to complete this process. This slide can also include the process used for analysis and synthesis of selected literature. A description of review matrices can be followed by an exemplar slide that includes a review table. Once the method has been clearly explained, the *results* will be included on the next slide. Begin this section with the *search flow diagram* that demonstrates what was retained and excluded in the review. Then, the *final results* slide will include results of the analysis and synthesis in bullet format. The next slide is the *discussion* slide. On this slide, the results are put in context and linked to what is known and what this review adds to the knowledge base. The final slide is the *conclusions and implications* slide where a discussion of the main findings of the review leads to recommendations for research, practice, and/or education and policy.

When the review is accepted for podium presentation, the conference organizers will designate the amount of time available for presentation. For most professional conferences, several individuals will present their work in a single session that may have a common theme. Most presentations are 10–15 minutes in length with 5 minutes for questions and answers. It is important to confirm the order of presentation and process that will be used when presenting. Many conferences will have room moderators who assist with loading the presentation onto the computer and keeping time for presenters. For some conferences, a speaker-ready room is available where the presenter loads the presentation onto the system and then confirms that the presentation is available when arriving to the presentation room. Sometimes a clock is available in the presentation room at the podium. The clock will start when the speaker begins and may flash to let the presenter know when the presentation should be completed. Presenters are encouraged to arrive to the presentation room 10–15 minutes in advance of the presentation to confirm processes, meet the room moderator, and verify presentation resources.

When presenting a podium presentation, it is important to keep the attention of the audience. Several factors enhance attention. First, slides should be readable from the back of the room. If attendees cannot see the slides or read the content on them, interest may be lost. Slides should have minimal information on them and be simple without a fancy graphics or distracting images. Simple PowerPoint slides with a light background and black letters may be easiest to read. Second, presenters should not simply read slides but instead summarize the points for the audience. Attendees can read the slides themselves if interested. Presenters should speak loudly, clearly, and face the audience rather than the presentation screen when speaking. Finally, presenters should practice the presentation to ensure adherence to the time allotted. For most conferences, the standard is 1 minute per slide in a podium presentation. In order to maintain this timing, practice will be required to stay within these guidelines.

7.3.3　Poster Presentation

Posters include the same headings as previously described for manuscripts and podium presentation of the findings of IRs. Posters differ in volume of content from journal articles due to space limitations. However, the content on the poster should provide the necessary information to convey the main review findings. When accepted for a poster presentation at a conference, presenters are notified about the size requirements of the poster. Posters are generally created using a poster template; the most common one is PowerPoint. If representing an organization, a poster template may be available for use through the organization. General rules for font sizes in poster presentations are: 85 point font for title, 56 point font for author(s) names and institutions, 36 point font for headings, and 24 point font for text. Text on the poster is left-justified using both upper and lowercase letters (Browner 2006). If a Sans Serif font like Arial or Helvetica is used for the text and titles, use a Serif-based font like Palatino or Times New Roman for figure legends or tables. It is not recommended that more than two fonts are used in creating a poster for presentation. Finally, begin the sections of the poster in the order in which they should be read from left to right starting at the top left panel.

The content included on poster panels follows the same format as those created for a podium presentation. The poster is usually divided into three main vertical panels with two or three sections per panel. Figure 7.5 is an example of a poster presentation. The introduction section (Sect. 7.1), found in the top left panel, includes the background of what is known about the topic of interest and the reason for completing the review. Bullet points are generally used to convey the main ideas with references to support the points made. The next panel, located on the left below the introduction section, is the purpose statement and any review questions (Sect. 7.2). The final panel on the left below the purpose statement is the method section. For the poster presentation, bullet points that identify keywords and databases searched as well as inclusion and exclusion criteria for search can be listed (Sect. 7.3). The criteria for appraising the quality of the literature are also included here as bullet points.

The top middle is the spot in the method section where the search flow diagram can be included to demonstrate decisions made about what literature was included and excluded from the review (Sect. 7.4). In the middle panel below the flow

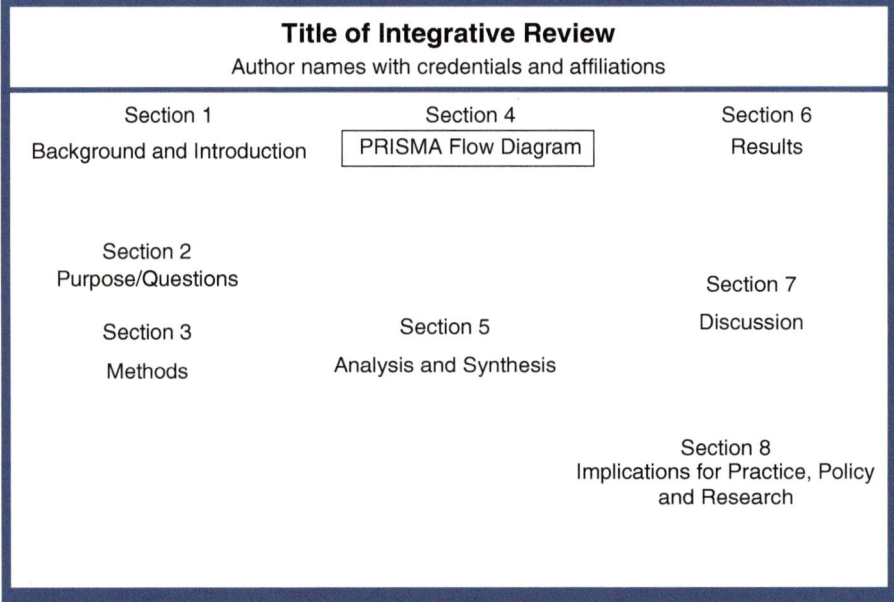

Fig. 7.5 Exemplar of a poster presentation for a conference

diagram, the analysis and synthesis of selected literature can be included by inserting the data tables, if there is room (Sect. 7.5). If there is inadequate room for the actual data tables, a description of the analysis and synthesis methods can be included.

The panel on the top right is where results will be presented (Sect. 7.6). A bulleted list of major findings includes the similarities and differences of the reviewed literature. The middle panel on the right below the results is the discussion section (Sect. 7.7). In this section, the reviewer will highlight the major findings of the study and link these findings to extant literature with the goal of highlighting what the review adds to the knowledge base. The final panel on the bottom right includes the implications for research, practice, and/or education and policy based on the findings of the review (Sect. 7.8). Due to space limitations, the abstract and references are not usually included on the poster and may be printed on a separate document and posted next to the poster for those who are interested.

The format of poster presentations varies by conference. In some instances, posters are displayed for the entire conference, and attendees can view them at any time throughout the conference. Presenters may only be present at the poster for a limited time to answer questions about the content. In other cases, posters may only be displayed for a predefined block of time during which poster presenters are available to answer any questions about the poster. In both cases, presenters should develop, in advance, a brief 1-minute summary that provides an overview of the main takeaway points of the poster for those who view it. Presenters should be present at the times assigned for presentation of the poster so interested participants can ask any questions. When accepted for poster presentation, the acceptance letter usually outlines the responsibilities of the poster presenter and includes the schedule for viewing times.

7.4 Submitting the Integrative Review for Publication

7.4.1 Selecting a Journal

There are several steps that must be taken prior to submitting a review for publication. First, select the appropriate journal for the topic of the review. Ideally, the intended journal should be selected prior to beginning the writing process, so that the review is written with the requirements and focus of that journal in mind. The focus of the review, emphasis of the targeted journal, intended audience for the review, and professional career goals of the reviewer guide the choice of journal (Collins et al. 2015; Balch et al. 2018). If there are coauthors, they should be consulted early in the process about which journal is the best fit for the topic of interest and also to determine the order of authors on the publication. If the focus of the review is to summarize the state of more clinically based research, then a clinically focused journal may be a good choice. For example, pediatric nurses who want to describe interventions to improve vaccination knowledge of parents may choose the *Journal of Pediatric Nursing*. However, if the purpose of the review is to summarize theoretical/conceptual work in a specific area, then a journal that is more theoretically oriented may be a better choice. For example, a pediatric nurse who wants to summarize theoretical models of vaccine decision making in parents of children may instead choose *Advances in Nursing Science*. This reiterates the idea that the focus of the review is important as a first step in the journal selection process.

The emphasis and audience for a journal can be determined by searching the author guidelines or *Instructions for Authors* section of a specific journal. To find these guidelines, enter the name of the journal followed by *Instructions for Authors* or *Guidelines for Authors* in the search. Frequently, a page of instructions for authors wishing to submit to a journal includes the purpose or mission of the journal, audience of the journal, and types of publications accepted by the journal. This can also be found at the beginning of published copies of the journal. In order to prevent rejection of the manuscript, it is important to review the mission and scope of the journal (Flanagan 2018). Table 7.1 provides an overview and comparison of two different journals as an exemplar of this process. Prospective authors can also review recent editions of the publication to determine whether IRs have been published by the journal. A search within the journal can also be done by entering the keyword integrative review within the journal search bar on the home page to quickly determine if this type of review has been published in the past. Potential authors may want to search in the same manner to determine if an IR that is similar to the topic has been recently published, since journals may not want another review on the same topic within a 3 to 5-year span of time. Finally, if a recent IR is not found in the journal, a query letter can be submitted to the editor of the journal describing the focus of the review. The name and contact information of the editor(s) of the journal can also

Table 7.1 Considerations of when choosing a journal for submission with exemplars

Characteristic	Definition of characteristic	Nursing research	Journal of pediatric nursing
Emphasis of the journal	The aims and scope of the journal found on the journal website or at the beginning of the paper journal	The editorial mission of *Nursing Research* is to report scientific research findings that advance understanding of all aspects of health. Research across the spectrum of biological, behavioral, psychosocial, and spiritual factors in health is published. Research that investigates links across scales of biosocial organization, from cells to society, is welcome. Nursing intervention and outcome research are critical aspects of the editorial focus of *Nursing Research*. Basic, translational, and clinical research is published	*The Journal of Pediatric Nursing: Nursing Care of Children and Families* is interested in publishing evidence-based practice, quality improvement, theory, and research papers on a variety of topics from United States and international authors. Journal content covers the life span from birth to adolescence. Submissions should be pertinent to the *nursing* care needs of healthy and ill infants, children, and adolescents, addressing their biopsychosocial needs
Impact factor	The average number of citations from a journal over the past 2 years that is cited in that year	Impact factor: 2.020	Impact factor: 1.563
Journal website	Link to information about the journal	https://www.journals.lww.com/nursingresearchonline/pages/default.aspx	https://www.journals.elsevier.com/journal-of-pediatric-nursing
Manuscript type	Types of manuscripts accepted by the journal. Described in the aims and scope section	*Nursing Research* publishes regular papers and brief reports in the following areas: Research Reports, Reviews, Methods, Brief Reports, Commentaries	*The Journal of Pediatric Nursing: Nursing Care of Children and Families (JPN)* is interested in publishing evidence-based practice, quality improvement, theory, and research papers on a variety of topics from United States and international authors. *JPN* also features the following regular columns for which authors may submit brief papers: Hot Topics and Technology

(continued)

Table 7.1 (continued)

Characteristic	Definition of characteristic	Nursing research	Journal of pediatric nursing
Word count or page limit	Guidelines provided by the journal about different types of articles accepted for publication and associated word counts. Found in the information for authors section	8–16 pages depending on type of paper	
Audience	The targeted audience for the journal described on the website	*Nursing Research* has been a "cooperative venture" of scientists, professional organizations, publisher, editorial staff, and readers to circulate scientific papers in nursing to improve care, alleviate suffering, and advance well-being. Today, *Nursing Research* continues as a preeminent journal in the field and is the official journal of the Eastern Nursing Research Society (ENRS) and the Western Institute of Nursing (WIN)	*JPN* is the official journal of the Society of Pediatric Nurses and the Pediatric Endocrinology Nursing Society

Place your letterhead here

Your name and credentials
Address
City, State

Date

Name of Editor
Name of journal
address of journal
City, State

Dear Editor:

I have completed writing an integrative review on heart failure symptoms and the relationship of those symptoms to delay in treatment seeking. The results suggest that the characteristics of symptoms influence treatment seeking delay. The title of the manuscript is XX. I believe this manuscript may be of importance to your readership based on the topic. I am inquiring about whether your journal publishes integrative review manuscripts. The authors all made contributions to the conception, design and writing of the manuscript. The work is currently not being considered at another journal.

Sincerely,

Your name and credentials
Email address

Fig. 7.6 Example of a query letter to an editor of a journal

generally be found in the *Information for Authors* or journal information home page. An example of a query letter is found in Fig. 7.6.

The final consideration prior to submitting an IR for publication is the author's own career goals. For many authors, their primary goal is to improve practice or advance science through publication. As a result, an author may want to publish in a journal affiliated with an organization that focuses on the topic of the review. For example, *Nursing Research* is the official journal of the Eastern Nursing Research Society. If an author publishes in this journal, the article will likely be read by members of this organization, thus increasing recognition among this membership. Knowledge of an author's scholarly work by others may be an important consideration during tenure and promotion processes; therefore, the selected journal is important. Another consideration for those seeking tenure or promotion within an institution is the type of journal selected for publication. Journals have different rankings that can be found in *Journal Citation Reports*. The journal rank is determined based on the number of citations of articles in that journal divided by the number of published articles over the past 2 years. The impact factor is the average number of citations from a journal over the past 2 years that is cited in that year (Garfield 2006). These factors may be used in tenure and promotion decisions and should be considered when deciding where to submit the review article for publication. Finally, the ability to reach a certain audience may be a goal of publication. Some authors may choose to pay an additional fee to publish their article in an open-access journal. Open-access journals charge the author a publication fee that can range in price. The publication fee allows the publisher to make the article available to everyone online rather than just those who subscribe to the journal. Authors may choose to pay this fee to increase the audience for their article. However, authors are cautioned to investigate the journal to be sure it is not considered a predatory journal. Predatory journals, also known as "pay-to-publish" journals, have inconsistent or nonexistent editing and publishing processes when compared to peer-reviewed journals (Milton 2019). Typically, peer review does not occur in these journals, thus lowering the quality of publications (Bourgault 2019). Finally, predatory journals may not be accessible or searchable through standard databases, thus limiting the ability of a review to be found by the intended audience.

7.4.2   Preparing the Manuscript for Submission

Once the primary author and any coauthors have agreed on the targeted journal, it will be important to review the *Information for Authors* or *Guidelines for Authors* section of the journal as described earlier. Review the requirements for publishing in the journal carefully, and follow them to prevent rejection of the manuscript by peer reviewers. Publishing guidelines include the specific format of the article (full length versus brief report), margin size, font size and type, page or word limitations, table and figure guidelines, references, abstract, title page, and keywords. Some publishers require authors to submit a PRISMA checklist with the manuscript. Many journals have word limits, often 4000–5000 words, but may be as high as 7000 words. In addition, many journals require authors to meet specific authorship guidelines and to confirm their role in the manuscript preparation process at submission. These guidelines may differ by journal; however, commonly accepted guidelines for authorship include substantial contributions to the conception, design, and writing of the paper; acquisition, interpretation, or analysis of the data; drafting or critical revision of the paper; and approval of the final article for submission (International Committee of Medical Journal Editors 2018).

Acknowledgment of those who assisted in manuscript preparation but do not qualify for full authorship status is another consideration described in the *Information for Authors* section. Be sure to have all authors review and confirm the final version of the IR manuscript prior to submission. Most journals will require some type of signed documentation from each author related to copyright and conflict of interest. Documentation may be required at the time of submission or upon article acceptance. It is recommended to read the author guidelines carefully.

7.4.3 Manuscript Submission and Review

7.4.3.1 Submission

Manuscript submission processes vary by publisher. Potential authors should review the steps for manuscript submission on the selected journal's website and carefully follow them. Generally, instructions for submission are written or found in a guided tutorial on the publisher's website with exemplars of required formatting of content. Most journals require online submission with uploading of supporting documents through a web-based portal. Authors need to register for an account with the journal in order to complete the submission process. Often one author will be designated the *Corresponding Author;* this is the person responsible for uploading the required documents and communicating with journal personnel. When determining order of authors at the beginning of the publication process, the *Corresponding Author* should be determined. This may or may not be the primary author of the review.

Documents required during manuscript submission may include a cover letter to the editor, manuscript, tables, figures, and a title page as separate documents. The cover letter allows the author to summarize the manuscript, outline the novelty of the review, and convince the editor that this is a topic worthy of publication in the selected journal. The title page is often submitted as a separate document to facilitate anonymity during the peer review process. Tables and figures are also generally submitted as separate documents since the publisher determines the placement of these in the final manuscript. Copyright and conflict of interest forms may be required at the time of submission. These forms are generally found on the publisher's website and should be completed by each author and uploaded at the time of submission. However, some publishers do not require submission of these forms until the manuscript has been accepted for publication. In this case, publishers may ask for the contact information for each coauthor and send the required forms directly to each coauthor.

If any figures, tables, or text includes content that has previously been published, permission to reproduce the content should be obtained from the copyright holder. In many cases, the copyright holder is the publisher of the journal in which the content is published, unless explicitly stated. In this case, permission to reproduce the content can often be obtained by completing a form found on the publisher's website that is submitted with other documents at the time of manuscript submission. To determine the policies and processes for obtaining permission to reuse content, search the copyright holder's website with the keyword copyright permission. Once the manuscript submission is complete, including copyrights and permissions, a confirmation email is sent to the *Corresponding Author*, and in some case coauthors, from the publisher confirming submission of the manuscript.

7.4.3.2 Manuscript Review

Once a review manuscript has been submitted for publication, it will be initially reviewed by the journal editor for compatibility with the format and content of the journal. If the manuscript meets basic requirements of this preliminary review, the editor will send it to two or three peer reviewers for full review. Some journals request that potential authors suggest peer reviewers for the review manuscript when it is submitted for publication. Authors can find potential reviewers by searching the topical area of the review in a database to see who has published in the topical area of the review previously. The reference list of the review can also be checked to determine potential peer reviewers. The author of the review does not contact potential peer reviewers directly but suggests names to the editor during the online submission process. The editor will then review the credentials of the potential peer reviewer and formally make the peer review request.

Peer review processes vary by journal. Typically, peer reviews will be completed within 1 to 2 months of manuscript submission. *Corresponding Authors* can monitor the status of the manuscript by signing into the journal website with the registration credentials created during submission. On the website, the author can click on the status of the submitted manuscript link on a pull-down menu and see the current status of the review. This format also differs by publisher, but all manuscript submission websites include links to monitor the status of the submitted manuscript.

Once peer reviews are complete, the editor will compile reviewers' written recommendations into one summary document and send them to the *Corresponding Author* with recommendations to Accept with major or minor edits or Reject. Carefully review the letter from the editor to confirm the status of the manuscript. New authors may mistakenly think a manuscript is rejected when in fact the editor is interested in publishing it with editing. Commonly, editors may send a message of interest in the manuscript with revision but not indicate its acceptance without reviewing a revised manuscript. An example of this type of feedback is included further:

> I have received the comments of the peer reviewers on your manuscript, and copies of the feedback are included below. The peer reviewers believe that your manuscript is of potential interest to our readers but feel that substantial revision would be necessary before the paper could be considered again for publication. If you are willing to revise the manuscript taking into consideration the suggestions of the peer reviewers, I will send the revised paper to the original reviewers for their appraisal.

Read reviewers' comments carefully, and respond to each point made within the designated time limit. Some journals require the use of track changes to indicate where changes were made in the document. All journals will require a letter outlining the changes made in the manuscript in a *response to reviewers'* document. It is helpful to copy the reviewers' actual comments into this document and then address each point in a polite and respectful manner. Peer reviewers volunteer to complete reviews out of a sense of duty to the profession; therefore, not all have the exact expertise in a specific topical area. As a result, reviewers may lack consensus about a review or fail to recognize the particular method used in the review therefore not detecting flaws in the chosen method (Edwards 2015). An example of reviewer feedback and response is included further:

> (Reviewer) Method section: The author(s) state: "It is unknown how much prior education about heart failure these patients had as this information was not collected". Not knowing if the participants have had any heart failure education is a limitation and should be acknowledged in the Limitations section.

(Author(s) Response) We have included a statement in the limitations section that acknowledges this limitation.

Once revisions are completed, the revised document(s) is submitted using the same processes as the initial submission. All revised documents are submitted along with the *response to reviewers'* document that clearly outlines changes made or rationale for not making a recommended change.

Although manuscripts are the most popular form of scholarly dissemination of reviews, attention to newer mechanisms of dissemination might expand the audience for the review findings and reach nonprofessional audiences appropriate for IRs.

7.5   New Approaches for Dissemination of Reviews

Reviewers may be familiar with dissemination of scholarship through more traditional routes including publication in peer-reviewed journal articles and presentations at professional conferences. However, in order to reach the largest audience and disseminate the results widely, new approaches to dissemination are necessary. Translation gaps exist due to lack of effective communication with stakeholders, policymakers, nonscientists, and the use of mainly passive approaches to dissemination (Brownson et al. 2018). This results in limited uptake of research findings in practice, currently reported to take 17 years before adoption (Westfall et al. 2007). The use of news media and social media may increase dissemination of review findings to professional and nonprofessional groups.

7.5.1   News Media

Television, radio, and newspapers provide researchers with direct access to stakeholders and policymakers. News media outlets want to present research that will gain attention and be of interest to their audience. Like peer reviewers for journals and conferences, news media outlets want a compelling and clear case for presenting research findings. Several factors make a story newsworthy: seriousness of the problem, human interest, timeliness, and conflict or controversy (Brownson et al. 2018). Integrative reviews have the potential to include all of these elements based on the potential volume of research reviewed, thus increasing the strength of potentially conclusive findings in an area. For reviewers choosing this method of dissemination, it is important to develop a single message in nontechnical language (Brownson et al. 2018). Most organizations have a public relations department with individuals trained to assist with writing press releases or policy briefs and trained to speak to the media. If choosing to write a press release, include the logo of the institution, date of the release, and a short headline depicting major findings. Summarize the findings in two to three paragraphs written for a lay audience. Communicate the most important ideas first and keep the writing simple. Many of the briefs written for news media can also be disseminated through social media including Twitter, Facebook, Research Gate, and LinkedIn.

7.5.2   Social Media

Social media is a "collection of web-based technologies that share a user-focused approach to design and functionality, where users can actively participate in content creation and editing through open collaboration between members of communities of practice" (Cheston et al. 2013, p. 893). According to this definition, social networking sites such as Twitter, Facebook, LinkedIn, and Research Gate qualify as social media. In contrast to most professional publications and presentations, social networking sites such as Twitter and Facebook encourage two-way communication, thus making it a strong possibility for collaborative review dissemination. In fact, a study testing the use of this modality as a mechanism for disseminating research evidence to health practitioners reported that 26.9% of participants used it for obtaining research evidence and 15% used it to disseminate research evidence (Tunnecliff et al. 2015). In another study, researchers compared the use of Facebook versus Twitter for delivery of educational content by clinical experts normally disseminated at a professional conference. The results demonstrated that 70% of participants reported using the education received via social media in practice (Maloney et al. 2015). In fact, researchers currently use social media to educate medical students, recruit for research studies, and provide consultations (Cheston et al. 2013; Tunnecliff et al. 2015; Corey et al. 2018). However, current guidelines and recommendations for review dissemination using this modality do not exist.

   Social media sites allow individuals with similar interests to follow each other. By following another individual, whether friend, celebrity, or fellow researcher, research can be shared among a network with similar interests. When a review is complete and published or presented, a link to the title of the work can be posted in a 140-word Tweet or with a link on Facebook, LinkedIn, or Research Gate, thus notifying the research and practice community of its existence. With Twitter and Facebook, followers can retweet or forward information to other network members. Because so many individuals currently use these social networks, large amounts of information can be shared rapidly, thus decreasing the time for translation of potentially powerful research findings. In the future, expect the use of these modalities for dissemination of reviews to increase.

7.6   Future Needs to Update the Integrative Review

Discourse about review methods has occurred since the 1980s in several disciplines. Despite this discourse, formal guidelines for completing IRs were inconsistent, resulting in confusion about names for reviews, methods for reviews, and lack of clarity about appraisal processes used when conducting reviews (Aveyard and Bradbury-Jones 2019). In this book, the authors attempt to clarify the IR process for those who may be interested in undertaking this method of knowledge generation, providing a snapshot of the current state of IRs. The present value of this method is the ability to use diverse forms of literature (research, theoretical, and methodological) to critically analyze and synthesize what is known to make recommendations for research, practice and/or education, and policy.

In the future, new review methods developed may result in the need to update existing reporting guidelines for reviews. Further, the rigor of the IR is enhanced by critical appraisal of diverse forms of evidence (Torraco 2016). As science grows, consistent and validated appraisal tools may be developed requiring updating of the IR method. Finally, the volume of the literature generated continues to grow rapidly and in forms not seen in the past. Traditional paper journals have been replaced with primarily online journals. Publications now occur in a number of web- and cloud-based forums not searchable in current databases. The format of publications has changed as well from more traditional research length papers to research briefs further increasing available literature to review. All of these factors converge to support the continual revision and updating of the IR method so that it will continue to be a viable method of knowledge generation for future clinicians, scholars, educators, and policymakers in the future.

References

Alspach JG (2017) Writing for publication 101: why the abstract is so important. Crit Care Nurse 37(4):12–15. https://doi.org/10.4037/ccn2017466

Aveyard H, Bradbury-Jones C (2019) An analysis of current practices in undertaking literature reviews in nursing: findings from a focused mapping review and synthesis. BMC Med Res Methodol 19(1):105. https://doi.org/10.1186/s12874-019-0751-7

Balch CM, McMasters KM, Klimberg VS, Pawlik TM, Posner MC, Roh M et al (2018) Steps to getting your manuscript published in a high-quality medical journal. Ann Surg Oncol 25(4):850–855. https://doi.org/10.1245/s10434-017-6320

Bougioukas KI, Bouras E, Apostolidou-Kiouti F, Kokkali S, Arvanitidou M, Haidich AB (2019) Reporting guidelines on how to write a complete and transparent abstract for overviews of systematic reviews of health care interventions. J Clin Epidemiol 106:70–79. https://doi.org/10.1016/j.jclinepi.2018.10.005

Bourgault AM (2019) Predatory journals: a potential threat to nursing practice and science. Crit Care Nurse 39(4):9–11. https://doi.org/10.4037/ccn2019529

Browner WS (2006) Publishing and presenting clinical research. Lippincott, Williams and Wilkins, Philadelphia, pp 144–150

Brownson RC, Eyler AA, Harris JK, Moore JB, Tabak RG (2018) Getting the word out: new approaches for disseminating public health science. J Public Health Manag Pract 24(2):102–111. https://doi.org/10.1097/PHH.0000000000000673

Cheston CC, Flickinger TE, Chisolm MS (2013) Social media use in medical education: a systematic review. Acad Med 88(6):893–901. https://doi.org/10.1097/ACM.0b013e31828ffc23

Collins KA, Brannan GD, Dogbey GY (2015) Research dissemination: guiding the novice researcher on the publication path. J Am Osteopath Assoc 115(5):324–330. https://doi.org/10.7556/jaoa.2015.063

Cooper HM, Hedges LV, Valentine JC (2009) The handbook of research synthesis and meta-analysis. Russell Sage, New York, NY

Corey KL, McCurry MK, Sethares KA, Bourbonniere M, Hirschman KB, Meghani SH (2018) Utilizing Internet-based recruitment and data collection to access different age groups of former family caregivers. Appl Nurs Res 44:82–87. https://doi.org/10.1016/j.apnr.2018.10.005

Coughlin MB, Sethares KA (2017) Chronic sorrow in parents of children with a chronic illness or disability: an integrative literature review. J Pediatr Nurs 37:108–116. https://doi.org/10.1016/j.pedn.2017.06.011

Edwards DJ (2015) Dissemination of research results: on the path to practice change. Can J Hosp Pharm 68(6):465–469. https://doi.org/10.4212/cjhp.v68i6.1503

Flanagan J (2018) Scholarly papers for a course versus those submitted for publication. Int J Nurs Knowl 29(3):145. https://doi.org/10.1111/2047-3095.12221

Fowler J (2015) Writing for publication: from staff nurse to nurse consultant. Br J Nurs 24(17):898. https://doi.org/10.3928/00220124-20190218-04

Freysteinson WM, Stankus JA (2019) The language of scholarship: how to write an abstract that tells a compelling story. J Contin Educ Nurs 50(3):107–108

Garfield E (2006) The history and meaning of the journal impact factor. JAMA 295(1):90–93. https://doi.org/10.1001/jama.295.1.90

Houde SC, Melillo KD (2002) Cardiovascular health and physical activity in older adults: an integrative review of research methodology and results. J Adv Nurs. 38(3):219–234

International Committee of Medical Journal Editors (2018) Recommendations for the conduct, reporting, editing, and publication of scholarly work in medical journals 2018 [cited 2019 23 Aug 19]. http://www.icmje.org/news-and-editorials/icmje-recommendations_annotated_dec18.pdf

Maloney S, Tunnecliff J, Morgan P, Gaida JE, Clearihan L, Sadasivan S et al (2015) Translating evidence into practice via social media: a mixed-methods study. J Med Internet Res 17(10):e242. https://doi.org/10.2196/jmir.4763

Merriam Webster Dictionary (n.d.). https://www.merriam-webster.com/dictionary/dissemination

Milton CL (2019) Predatory publishing in nursing. Nurs Sci Q 32(3):180–181. https://doi.org/10.1177/2F0894318419845400

Moher D, Liberati A, Tetzlaff J, Altman DG, Group P (2009) Preferred reporting items for systematic reviews and meta-analyses: the PRISMA statement. Ann Intern Med 151(4):264–269. https://doi.org/10.1371/journal.pmed.1000097

Oermann MH, Hayes JC (2016) Writing for publication in nursing, 3rd edn. Springer, New York

Oermann MH, Christenbery T, Turner KM (2018) Writing publishable review, research, quality improvement, and evidence-based practice manuscripts. Nursing Economics 36(6):7

Sethares KA, Chin E, Jurgens CY (2015) Predictors of delay in heart failure patients and consequences for outcomes. Curr Heart Fail Rep 12(1):94–105. https://doi.org/10.1007/s11897-014-0241-5

Sturgeon CM, Ditadi A (2018) Let me speak! A reviewers' guide to writing a successful meeting abstract. Stem Cell Rep 11(6):1324–1326. https://doi.org/10.1016/j.stemcr.2018.11.016

Toronto CE, LaRocco SA (2019) Family perception of and experience with family presence during cardiopulmonary resuscitation: an integrative review. J Clin Nurs 28(1-2):32–46. https://doi.org/10.1177/0193945919845649

Torraco RJ (2016) Writing integrative literature reviews: using the past and present to explore the future. Hum Resour Dev Rev 15(4):404–428. https://doi.org/10.1177/1534484316671606

Tunnecliff J, Ilic D, Morgan P, Keating J, Gaida JE, Clearihan L et al (2015) The acceptability among health researchers and clinicians of social media to translate research evidence to clinical practice: mixed-methods survey and interview study. J Med Internet Res 17(5):e119. https://doi.org/10.2196/jmir.4347

Viveiros J, Chamberlain B, O'Hair A, Sethares K (2019) Mindfulness-based interventions in the heart failure population: an integrative review. Nurs Res 68(2):E135–EE 6. https://doi.org/10.1177/1474515119863181

Westfall JM, Mold J, Fagnan L (2007) Practice-based research—"Blue Highways" on the NIH roadmap. JAMA 297(4):403–406. https://doi.org/10.1001/jama.297.4.403

Whittemore R, Knafl K (2005) The integrative review: updated methodology. J Adv Nurs 52(5):546–553. https://doi.org/10.1111/j.1365-2648.2005.03621.x